The Complete Low Fiber Cookbook For Beginners

1500 Days of Delicious and Healthy Low Residue (Low Fiber) recipes for people with Diverticulitis, Ulcerative Colitis, IBD, and Crohn's Disease. Includes a 30 Day Meal Plan

Kathleen H. Jensen

CONTENTS

SALADS

MAIN DISHES

SIDES

SNACKS

DESERTS

Introduction

Understanding a Low Fiber Diet

A low-fiber diet is often recommended for specific health conditions or as a temporary measure to improve gastrointestinal comfort. What does this dietary approach involve, and who benefits the most from it?

This introductory chapter introduces you to the world of low-fiber cooking. We will start by explaining the concept of a low-fiber diet, discussing its importance, and examining its potential benefits and difficulties. Having a solid understanding will help you make informed dietary choices that can improve your well-being and overall quality of life.

What is a low-fiber diet?

A low-fiber diet is a nutritional strategy that involves limiting the intake of high-fiber foods. Fiber is the non-digestible part of plant-based foods, including fruits, vegetables, whole grains, and legumes. It is an essential component of a balanced diet, as it supports digestive health, aids in maintaining a healthy weight, and may lower the risk of chronic diseases. However, certain medical conditions and circumstances may require a temporary decrease in fiber consumption.

A low-fiber diet restricts the intake of foods that are high in fiber to reduce gastrointestinal discomfort, address certain health conditions, or prepare for medical procedures. While this may sound limiting, it is a feasible and sometimes temporary change intended to accomplish specific health goals.

Who should follow a low-fiber diet?

The suitability of a low fiber diet varies from person to person, primarily depending on their individual health needs and medical recommendations. It is commonly prescribed for individuals dealing with specific conditions, such as:

Gastrointestinal Disorders: Individuals with conditions such as Crohn's disease, diverticulitis, or bowel obstructions may find it helpful to follow a low-fiber diet during flare-ups or to promote healing.

Preoperative Preparation: Patients undergoing certain medical procedures, such as colonoscopy or bowel surgery, may be instructed to follow a low-fiber diet to achieve the best possible outcomes and reduce the risk of complications.

Postoperative Recovery: After certain surgeries, including gastrointestinal procedures, a low-fiber diet may be recommended to minimize strain on the digestive system during the initial stages of recovery.

Benefits of a Low Fiber Diet

A low-fiber diet, when correctly implemented under the guidance of a healthcare professional or dietitian, may provide several benefits:

Reduced fiber intake can minimize symptoms like bloating, cramping, and diarrhea in individuals with certain digestive disorders, resulting in increased gastrointestinal comfort.

Preparation for Medical Procedures: A low-fiber diet can help promote a clean and clear digestive tract, which is vital for effective medical procedures such as colonoscopies.

Postoperative Relief: After surgery, a low-fiber diet may be recommended to reduce strain on the gastrointestinal system and minimize potential complications associated with consuming high-fiber foods.

However, it's important to acknowledge that a low-fiber diet, while advantageous in certain circumstances, is generally not recommended for long-term use in most cases. There can be downsides to it, such as the possibility of experiencing nutritional deficiencies and having a limited range of food options.

The following chapters will explore the intricacies of planning and following a low-fiber diet. You'll find balanced meal plans and delicious recipes that cater to your dietary needs, providing you with the tools and inspiration to adopt this eating approach while prioritizing your health and well-being.

Chapter 1

Planning Your Low-Fiber Diet

Now that we have a basic understanding of what a low-fiber diet involves and who can benefit from it, the next important step is to plan your diet. Whether you're navigating this path due to a medical condition or preparing for a procedure, thoughtful and well-informed planning is vital to ensure that you maintain good nutrition, prevent deficiencies, and manage your symptoms effectively.

This chapter provides detailed information on planning a low-fiber diet, explaining the necessary steps to create a balanced meal plan. We'll discuss the importance of consulting with a healthcare professional or dietitian, provide tips for grocery shopping, and help you gain the knowledge needed to create a personalized dietary regimen that suits your specific needs and preferences.

Seeking advice from a dietitian.

One of the first and most essential steps in starting a low-fiber diet is to seek guidance from a registered dietitian or healthcare professional. Their expertise is valuable in tailoring a dietary plan to your health requirements. Here's what you can expect during this consultation:

Assessment of Medical Needs: Your dietitian will assess your medical history, specific condition, and any dietary restrictions to determine the appropriate level of fiber restriction and the diet duration.

Personalized Meal Planning: With their knowledge and experience, a dietitian will create a customized meal plan that ensures you receive the necessary nutrients while considering your dietary fiber intake. This plan will consider your preferences, allergies, and any other dietary restrictions you may have.

Monitoring and Adjustments: Your dietitian will monitor your health and make necessary adjustments to your low-fiber diet as you continue with it. If there is a risk of nutrient deficiencies, they may also suggest supplements.

Dietitians offer education and support by providing information about food choices and portion sizes, which helps you make informed decisions. They can also offer emotional support and guidance, which can be helpful during difficult dietary transitions.

Creating a meal plan.

After consulting with a dietitian and receiving a personalized plan, it is time to begin meal planning. Here are some essential factors to consider:

Balanced Nutrition: Your meal plan should provide you with all the necessary nutrients while also considering any restrictions on fiber intake. This includes vitamins, minerals, protein, and fats.

Portion Control: Managing portion sizes is critical to help prevent overeating and support healthy digestion. Your dietitian can provide personalized guidelines based on your specific needs.

Eat Variety: Incorporating various foods can help prevent dietary monotony and ensure you receive a wide range of nutrients. Please explore different low-fiber options within your prescribed limitations.

Follow a Meal Schedule: Stick to a regular meal schedule, which can help regulate digestion and potentially prevent discomfort. Skipping meals or irregular eating patterns may exacerbate gastrointestinal symptoms.

Fluid Intake: Adequate hydration is critical. Staying hydrated by drinking enough fluids can help reduce the risk of constipation and support overall health. Make sure you drink enough fluids throughout the day.

Tips for Grocery Shopping

Navigating the grocery store can be challenging when following a low-fiber diet. These tips can assist you in making informed choices and ensuring that your pantry is adequately stocked with suitable foods.

Read food labels: Make sure to carefully examine food labels to determine the amount of fiber they contain. Search for products that are specifically labeled as "**low fiber**" or "**fiber-restricted.**"

Stick to Your List: Create a shopping list based on your meal plan, and make sure to only purchase the items on the list. This helps avoid spontaneous purchases that may not align with your dietary requirements.

Shop the Perimeter: In most grocery stores, fresh produce and meats are usually found around the perimeter. Focus your shopping in these areas, as they often contain options with lower fiber content.

Consider Convenience: Pre-packaged, canned, or frozen low-fiber options can be convenient and save preparation time. Please be aware of additives and preservatives, and choose products that have undergone minimal processing.

Stock Up on Pantry Staples: Maintain a supply of low-fiber staples such as white rice, refined pasta, canned fruits and vegetables, and lean meats. This ensures you have the basics for creating various dishes with low fiber content.

Planning your low-fiber diet can be vital to managing your health effectively. By working closely with a dietitian, creating a balanced meal plan, and becoming a smart shopper, you'll be well-prepared to enjoy the recipes in the subsequent chapters of this cookbook. Together, we'll explore a diverse range of delicious recipes suitable for a low-fiber lifestyle.

BREAKFAST

Quinoa Breakfast Bowl with Berries

Prep Time: 10 minutes
Cook Time: 15 minutes
Number of Servings: 2

Ingredients:

- 1 cup quinoa

- 2 cups unsweetened almond milk

- 1/2 cup mixed berries (blueberries, strawberries, raspberries)

- 1/4 cup chopped nuts (almonds or walnuts)

- 1 tablespoon honey (optional)

- 1/2 teaspoon ground cinnamon

- 1/4 teaspoon vanilla extract

- 1/8 teaspoon iodized sea salt

Instructions:

1. Rinse the quinoa thoroughly in a fine-mesh strainer under cold running water.

2. In a medium saucepan, add the rinsed quinoa and almond milk. Bring to a boil over medium-high heat.

3. Reduce the heat to low, cover, and simmer for about 12-15 minutes, or until the quinoa is cooked and the liquid is absorbed. Stir occasionally to prevent sticking.

4. While the quinoa is cooking, prepare your mixed berries by washing them and slicing any larger fruits.

5. In a small bowl, add the mixed berries, chopped nuts, honey (if using), ground cinnamon, vanilla extract, and iodized sea salt. Mix sufficiently.

6. Once the quinoa is cooked, fluff it with a fork and divide it between two bowls.

7. Top each bowl of quinoa with the mixed berry and nut mixture.

8. Serve the quinoa breakfast bowls warm and enjoy your thyroid reset-friendly meal.

Nutritional Information (Per Serving):

- Carbs: 45 grams

- Fats: 12 grams

- Protein: 8 grams

- Sodium: 225 milligrams

Sweet Potato and Spinach Breakfast Skillet

Prep Time: 10 minutes
Cook Time: 20 minutes
Number of Servings: 2

Ingredients:

- 2 medium sweet potatoes, peeled and diced

- 1/2 onion, diced

- 2 cloves garlic, minced

- 2 cups fresh spinach leaves

- 4 large eggs

- 2 tablespoons olive oil

- 1/2 teaspoon iodized sea salt

- 1/4 teaspoon black pepper

- 1/4 teaspoon paprika (optional)

- Chopped fresh parsley for garnish (optional)

Instructions:

1. In a large skillet, heat the olive oil over medium heat.

2. Add the diced sweet potatoes and diced onion to the skillet. Cook for about 10 minutes, stirring occasionally, until the sweet potatoes are tender and lightly browned.

3. Add the minced garlic to the skillet and cook for an extra 1-2 minutes, until fragrant.

4. Stir in the fresh spinach leaves and cook for another 2-3 minutes, or until the spinach wilts and reduces in size.

5. Create four small wells in the mixture with a spoon. Crack one egg into each well.

6. Cover the skillet and cook for 4-5 minutes, or until the egg whites are set, but the yolks are still slightly runny. You can cook them longer if you prefer firmer yolks.

7. Season the entire skillet with iodized sea salt, black pepper, and paprika (if using).

8. Garnish with chopped fresh parsley if desired.

9. Serve the Sweet Potato and Spinach Breakfast Skillet hot, dividing it into two portions.

Nutritional Information (Per Serving):

- Carbs: 38 grams

- Fats: 18 grams

- Protein: 15 grams

- Sodium: 445 milligrams

Green Smoothie Bowl with Almond Butter

Prep Time: 10 minutes
Cook Time: 0 minutes
Number of Servings: 2

Ingredients:

- 2 cups fresh spinach leaves

- 1 ripe banana, peeled and sliced

- 1/2 avocado, peeled and pitted

- 1 cup unsweetened almond milk

- 2 tablespoons almond butter

- 1 tablespoon chia seeds

- 1 tablespoon honey (optional)

- 1/2 teaspoon iodized sea salt
- Sliced fresh fruit, nuts, and seeds for topping (e.g., berries, sliced banana, almonds, chia seeds)

Instructions:

1. In a blender, add the fresh spinach leaves, sliced banana, avocado, almond milk, almond butter, chia seeds, honey (if using), and iodized sea salt.

2. Blend until the mixture is smooth and creamy. If it's too thick, you can add more almond milk to reach your desired consistency.

3. Pour the green smoothie mixture into two bowls.

4. Top each bowl with sliced fresh fruit, nuts, and seeds according to your preference. Common choices include berries, sliced banana, almonds, and additional chia seeds.

5. Serve the Green Smoothie Bowl with Almond Butter immediately.

Nutritional Information (Per Serving):

- Carbs: 35 grams
- Fats: 20 grams
- Protein: 7 grams
- Sodium: 345 milligrams

Cinnamon Oatmeal with Walnuts

Prep Time: 5 minutes
Cook Time: 10 minutes
Number of Servings: 2

Ingredients:

- 1 cup rolled oats
- 2 cups water
- 1/2 teaspoon ground cinnamon
- 1/4 cup chopped walnuts
- 2 tablespoons honey (optional)

- 1/2 teaspoon iodized sea salt

Instructions:

1. In a saucepan, add the rolled oats and water.

2. Bring the mixture to a boil over medium heat.

3. Reduce the heat to low and add the ground cinnamon, chopped walnuts, honey (if using), and iodized sea salt. Stir sufficiently to combine.

4. Simmer the oatmeal for about 5-7 minutes, stirring occasionally, until it reaches your desired consistency. If it becomes too thick, you can add a bit more water.

5. Take out the saucepan from the heat.

6. Divide the Cinnamon Oatmeal with Walnuts into two bowls.

7. You can drizzle a little more honey on top if desired.

8. Serve the oatmeal hot, and enjoy your thyroid reset-friendly meal.

Nutritional Information (Per Serving):

- Carbs: 34 grams

- Fats: 11 grams

- Protein: 6 grams

- Sodium: 250 milligrams

Chia Seed Pudding with Mango
Prep Time: 10 minutes (plus overnight chilling)
Cook Time: 0 minutes
Number of Servings: 2

Ingredients:

- 1/4 cup chia seeds

- 1 cup unsweetened almond milk

- 1 ripe mango, peeled, pitted, and diced

- 1 tablespoon honey (optional)

- 1/2 teaspoon iodized sea salt
- Sliced almonds for garnish (optional)

Instructions:

1. In a bowl, add the chia seeds and unsweetened almond milk. Mix sufficiently to ensure the chia seeds are evenly distributed in the liquid.

2. Cover the bowl and refrigerate the mixture for at least 4 hours or overnight. This allows the chia seeds to absorb the liquid and create a pudding-like texture.

3. Once the chia pudding has set, give it a good stir.

4. In a separate bowl, mix the diced ripe mango with honey (if using) and iodized sea salt.

5. Divide the chia seed pudding between two serving dishes.

6. Top each portion with the mango mixture.

7. If desired, garnish with sliced almonds.

8. Serve the Chia Seed Pudding with Mango chilled and enjoy your thyroid reset-friendly dessert or breakfast.

Nutritional Information (Per Serving):

- Carbs: 35 grams
- Fats: 10 grams
- Protein: 5 grams
- Sodium: 245 milligrams

Veggie Breakfast Tacos with Avocado

Prep Time: 15 minutes
Cook Time: 15 minutes
Number of Servings: 2

Ingredients:

- 4 small whole-grain tortillas
- 1 cup diced bell peppers (a mix of red, green, and yellow)

- 1/2 cup diced red onion
- 1 cup sliced mushrooms
- 1 cup baby spinach leaves
- 4 large eggs
- 1 ripe avocado, sliced
- 1 tablespoon olive oil
- 1/2 teaspoon iodized sea salt
- 1/4 teaspoon black pepper
- 1/4 teaspoon paprika (optional)
- Salsa for garnish (optional)
- Fresh cilantro leaves for garnish (optional)

Instructions:

1. In a large skillet, heat the olive oil over medium heat.
2. Add the diced bell peppers, diced red onion, and sliced mushrooms to the skillet. Cook for about 5 minutes, or until the vegetables are tender.
3. Stir in the baby spinach leaves and cook for an extra 2 minutes, or until they wilt.
4. Push the cooked vegetables to one side of the skillet, creating space for the eggs.
5. Crack the four eggs into the empty side of the skillet. Cook the eggs to your desired level of doneness, whether you prefer them scrambled or fried.
6. Season the entire skillet with iodized sea salt, black pepper, and paprika (if using).
7. Warm the whole-grain tortillas in a dry skillet or microwave according to the package instructions.
8. Divide the cooked vegetable and egg mixture between the tortillas.
9. Top each taco with slices of ripe avocado.
10. If desired, garnish with salsa and fresh cilantro leaves.

11. Serve the Veggie Breakfast Tacos with Avocado hot and enjoy your thyroid reset-friendly meal.

Nutritional Information (Per Serving):

- Carbs: 40 grams

- Fats: 22 grams

- Protein: 17 grams

- Sodium: 580 milligrams

Pumpkin Spice Overnight Oats

Prep Time: 10 minutes (plus overnight chilling)
Cook Time: 0 minutes
Number of Servings: 2

Ingredients:

- 1 cup rolled oats

- 1 1/2 cups unsweetened almond milk

- 1/2 cup canned pumpkin puree

- 2 tablespoons pure maple syrup

- 1 teaspoon ground cinnamon

- 1/4 teaspoon ground nutmeg

- 1/4 teaspoon ground ginger

- 1/4 teaspoon iodized sea salt

- 1/4 cup chopped pecans

- 1/4 cup dried cranberries

Instructions:

1. In a bowl, add the rolled oats, unsweetened almond milk, canned pumpkin puree, pure maple syrup, ground cinnamon, ground nutmeg, ground ginger, and iodized sea salt. Mix sufficiently to ensure all ingredients are thoroughly combined.

2. Cover the bowl and refrigerate the mixture for at least 4 hours or overnight. This allows the oats to absorb the liquid and develop a creamy texture.

3. Before serving, give the Pumpkin Spice Overnight Oats a good stir.

4. Divide the oat mixture between two serving bowls.

5. Top each bowl with chopped pecans and dried cranberries.

6. If desired, drizzle a little extra maple syrup on top for added sweetness.

7. Serve the Pumpkin Spice Overnight Oats cold or at room temperature and enjoy your thyroid reset-friendly breakfast.

Nutritional Information (Per Serving):

- Carbs: 53 grams

- Fats: 16 grams

- Protein: 7 grams

- Sodium: 375 milligrams

Broccoli and Feta Breakfast Muffins

Prep Time: 15 minutes
Cook Time: 25 minutes
Number of Servings: 6 muffins

Ingredients:

- 1 cup broccoli florets, finely chopped

- 1/2 cup crumbled feta cheese

- 1/4 cup diced red bell pepper

- 1/4 cup diced red onion

- 4 large eggs

- 1/4 cup unsweetened almond milk

- 1/4 cup oat flour

- 1/2 teaspoon baking powder

- 1/4 teaspoon iodized sea salt
- 1/4 teaspoon black pepper
- 1/4 teaspoon dried oregano
- Cooking spray or olive oil for greasing

Instructions:

1. Turn on your oven and set it to 350°F (175°C) to preheat. Grease a muffin tin with cooking spray or a light coating of olive oil.

2. In a large mixing bowl, add the finely chopped broccoli florets, crumbled feta cheese, diced red bell pepper, and diced red onion. Mix them together evenly.

3. In a separate bowl, whisk the large eggs and unsweetened almond milk until well combined.

4. Add the oat flour, baking powder, iodized sea salt, black pepper, and dried oregano to the egg mixture. Stir until you have a smooth batter.

5. Pour the egg batter over the broccoli and feta mixture. Stir everything together until all ingredients are well incorporated.

6. Divide the mixture into 6 muffin cups, filling each one almost to the top.

7. Bake in the preheated oven for approximately 25 minutes or until the muffins are set and the tops are lightly golden brown.

8. Take out the muffins from the oven and let them cool in the muffin tin for a few minutes.

9. Use a knife or spatula to gently lift the muffins out of the tin and onto a wire rack to cool completely.

10. Once cooled, the Broccoli and Feta Breakfast Muffins are ready to serve. Enjoy your thyroid reset-friendly breakfast!

Nutritional Information (Per Muffin):

- Carbs: 6 grams
- Fats: 7 grams
- Protein: 8 grams

- Sodium: 320 milligrams

Pumpkin Spice Chia Pudding

Prep Time: 10 minutes (plus overnight chilling)
Cook Time: 0 minutes
Number of Servings: 2

Ingredients:

- 1/4 cup chia seeds
- 1 1/2 cups unsweetened almond milk
- 1/2 cup canned pumpkin puree
- 2 tablespoons pure maple syrup
- 1/2 teaspoon ground cinnamon
- 1/4 teaspoon ground nutmeg
- 1/4 teaspoon ground ginger
- 1/4 teaspoon iodized sea salt
- 1/4 cup chopped walnuts
- 1/4 cup dried cranberries

Instructions:

1. In a bowl, add the chia seeds and unsweetened almond milk. Stir sufficiently to ensure the chia seeds are evenly distributed in the liquid.

2. Add the canned pumpkin puree, pure maple syrup, ground cinnamon, ground nutmeg, ground ginger, and iodized sea salt to the chia mixture. Mix thoroughly to incorporate all the ingredients.

3. Cover the bowl and refrigerate the Pumpkin Spice Chia Pudding for at least 4 hours or overnight. This allows the chia seeds to absorb the liquid and create a pudding-like consistency.

4. Before serving, give the chia pudding a good stir to make sure the ingredients are well combined.

5. Divide the pudding into two serving bowls.

6. Top each bowl with chopped walnuts and dried cranberries.

7. If desired, drizzle a bit of extra maple syrup on top for added sweetness.

8. Serve the Pumpkin Spice Chia Pudding cold or at room temperature and enjoy your thyroid reset-friendly dessert or breakfast.

Nutritional Information (Per Serving):

- Carbs: 45 grams

- Fats: 15 grams

- Protein: 6 grams

- Sodium: 340 milligrams

Spinach and Mushroom Breakfast Casserole Pudding

Prep Time: 15 minutes
Cook Time: 45 minutes
Number of Servings: 4

Ingredients:

- 8 large eggs

- 1 1/2 cups unsweetened almond milk

- 2 cups fresh spinach leaves, chopped

- 1 cup sliced mushrooms

- 1/2 cup diced red bell pepper

- 1/2 cup diced red onion

- 1/2 teaspoon iodized sea salt

- 1/4 teaspoon black pepper

- 1/4 teaspoon dried thyme

- Cooking spray or olive oil for greasing

Instructions:

1. Turn on your oven and set it to 350°F (175°C) to preheat. Grease a baking dish with cooking spray or a light coating of olive oil.

2. In a large mixing bowl, whisk the large eggs and unsweetened almond milk until well combined.

3. Add the chopped fresh spinach leaves, sliced mushrooms, diced red bell pepper, and diced red onion to the egg mixture. Stir until all ingredients are evenly distributed.

4. Season the mixture with iodized sea salt, black pepper, and dried thyme. Mix sufficiently.

5. Pour the spinach and mushroom mixture into the greased baking dish, spreading it evenly.

6. Bake in the preheated oven for approximately 45 minutes or until the casserole is set, and the top is lightly golden brown.

7. Take out the casserole from the oven and let it cool for a few minutes before slicing it into servings.

8. Serve the Spinach and Mushroom Breakfast Casserole Pudding warm, and enjoy your thyroid reset-friendly breakfast.

Nutritional Information (Per Serving):

- Carbs: 8 grams

- Fats: 14 grams

- Protein: 12 grams

- Sodium: 490 milligrams

Coconut Flour Waffles with Mixed Berry Compote

Prep Time: 15 minutes
Cook Time: 15 minutes
Number of Servings: 4

Ingredients:

For the Coconut Flour Waffles:

- 1/2 cup coconut flour

- 1/2 teaspoon baking powder

- 1/4 teaspoon iodized sea salt

- 4 large eggs

- 1 cup unsweetened almond milk
- 2 tablespoons coconut oil, melted
- 2 tablespoons pure maple syrup
- 1/2 teaspoon vanilla extract

For the Mixed Berry Compote:

- 1 cup mixed berries (blueberries, strawberries, raspberries)
- 1 tablespoon pure maple syrup
- 1/4 teaspoon iodized sea salt
- 1/4 teaspoon ground cinnamon
- 1/4 teaspoon vanilla extract

Instructions:

For the Coconut Flour Waffles:

1. Preheat your waffle iron according to the manufacturer's instructions.
2. In a mixing bowl, add the coconut flour, baking powder, and iodized sea salt.
3. In a separate bowl, whisk the large eggs, unsweetened almond milk, melted coconut oil, pure maple syrup, and vanilla extract.
4. Pour the wet ingredients into the dry ingredients and stir until a smooth batter forms. Let the batter rest for a couple of minutes to allow the coconut flour to absorb some of the liquid.
5. Lightly grease the waffle iron with a small amount of coconut oil or non-stick cooking spray.
6. Pour enough batter into the preheated waffle iron to cover the waffle grid, then close the lid.
7. Cook the waffles according to your waffle iron's instructions, typically for about 3-5 minutes, or until golden brown and crisp.
8. Carefully take out the waffles from the iron and keep them warm while you prepare the mixed berry compote.

For the Mixed Berry Compote:

1. In a small saucepan, add the mixed berries, pure maple syrup, iodized sea salt, ground cinnamon, and vanilla extract.

2. Cook the mixture over medium heat, stirring occasionally, for about 5 minutes, or until the berries have softened and released their juices.

3. Use the back of a spoon to lightly crush some of the berries to create a thicker compote consistency.

4. Take out the saucepan from heat.

5. Serve the Coconut Flour Waffles warm, topped with the Mixed Berry Compote.

Nutritional Information (Per Serving - 2 Waffles with Compote):

- Carbs: 26 grams

- Fats: 13 grams

- Protein: 9 grams

- Sodium: 425 milligrams

Turmeric and Ginger Oatmeal

Prep Time: 5 minutes
Cook Time: 10 minutes
Number of Servings: 2

Ingredients:

- 1 cup rolled oats

- 2 cups unsweetened almond milk

- 1/2 teaspoon ground turmeric

- 1/2 teaspoon ground ginger

- 1/4 teaspoon iodized sea salt

- 1/4 teaspoon black pepper

- 2 tablespoons honey (optional)

- 1/4 cup chopped almonds

- 1/4 cup diced dried apricots

- 1/4 cup unsweetened shredded coconut

Instructions:

1. In a saucepan, add the rolled oats and unsweetened almond milk.

2. Add the ground turmeric, ground ginger, iodized sea salt, and black pepper to the saucepan. Stir sufficiently to combine.

3. Place the saucepan over medium heat and bring the mixture to a simmer.

4. Reduce the heat to low and let the oatmeal simmer for about 5-7 minutes, stirring occasionally, or until it reaches your desired thickness and the oats are cooked.

5. If desired, add honey for sweetness and stir until it's fully incorporated.

6. In the meantime, toast the chopped almonds in a dry skillet over medium heat for 2-3 minutes or until they become fragrant and lightly golden. Take them out from the heat and set aside.

7. Serve the Turmeric and Ginger Oatmeal hot, dividing it between two bowls.

8. Top each bowl with toasted chopped almonds, diced dried apricots, and unsweetened shredded coconut.

Nutritional Information (Per Serving):

- Carbs: 54 grams

- Fats: 16 grams

- Protein: 11 grams

- Sodium: 285 milligrams

Broccoli and Smoked Salmon Egg Muffins

Prep Time: 10 minutes
Cook Time: 20 minutes
Number of Servings: 6

Ingredients:

- 6 large eggs

- 1/4 cup unsweetened almond milk
- 1 cup broccoli florets, finely chopped
- 3 ounces smoked salmon, diced
- 1/4 cup diced red onion
- 1/4 teaspoon iodized sea salt
- 1/4 teaspoon black pepper
- 1/4 teaspoon dried dill
- Cooking spray or olive oil for greasing

Instructions:

1. Turn on your oven and set it to 350°F (175°C) to preheat. Grease a muffin tin with cooking spray or a light coating of olive oil.

2. In a mixing bowl, whisk the large eggs and unsweetened almond milk until well combined.

3. Add the finely chopped broccoli florets, diced smoked salmon, diced red onion, iodized sea salt, black pepper, and dried dill to the egg mixture. Stir until all ingredients are evenly distributed.

4. Carefully pour the mixture into the greased muffin tin, dividing it equally among the cups.

5. Place the muffin tin in the preheated oven and bake for approximately 18-20 minutes or until the egg muffins are set and the tops are lightly golden brown.

6. Take out the muffin tin from the oven and let it cool for a few minutes.

7. Use a knife or spatula to gently lift the egg muffins out of the tin and onto a serving plate.

8. Serve the Broccoli and Smoked Salmon Egg Muffins warm, and enjoy your thyroid reset-friendly breakfast.

Nutritional Information (Per Serving - 1 Egg Muffin):

- Carbs: 1 gram
- Fats: 6 grams
- Protein: 7 grams

- Sodium: 230 milligrams

Turmeric and Ginger Breakfast Quinoa Bowl
Prep Time: 5 minutes
Cook Time: 15 minutes
Number of Servings: 2

Ingredients:

- 1 cup quinoa

- 2 cups unsweetened almond milk

- 1/2 teaspoon ground turmeric

- 1/2 teaspoon ground ginger

- 1/4 teaspoon iodized sea salt

- 1/4 teaspoon black pepper

- 2 tablespoons honey (optional)

- 1/4 cup sliced almonds

- 1/4 cup dried cranberries

- 1/4 cup diced dried apricots

Instructions:

1. Rinse the quinoa thoroughly under cold running water using a fine-mesh sieve.

2. In a saucepan, add the rinsed quinoa and unsweetened almond milk.

3. Add the ground turmeric, ground ginger, iodized sea salt, and black pepper to the saucepan. Stir sufficiently to combine.

4. Place the saucepan over medium-high heat and bring the mixture to a boil.

5. Reduce the heat to low, cover the saucepan, and let the quinoa simmer for approximately 12-15 minutes, or until it's cooked and most of the liquid is absorbed. Stir occasionally.

6. If desired, drizzle honey over the cooked quinoa and mix sufficiently.

7. Divide the Turmeric and Ginger Breakfast Quinoa between two serving bowls.

8. Top each bowl with sliced almonds, dried cranberries, and diced dried apricots.

9. Serve the breakfast quinoa hot and enjoy your thyroid reset-friendly meal.

Nutritional Information (Per Serving):

- Carbs: 65 grams

- Fats: 12 grams

- Protein: 11 grams

- Sodium: 300 milligrams

Spinach and Feta Egg White Omelette

Prep Time: 5 minutes
Cook Time: 10 minutes
Number of Servings: 1

Ingredients:

- 3 large egg whites

- 1 cup fresh spinach leaves, chopped

- 1/4 cup crumbled feta cheese

- 1/4 cup diced red onion

- 1/4 teaspoon iodized sea salt

- 1/4 teaspoon black pepper

- Cooking spray or olive oil for greasing

Instructions:

1. In a bowl, whisk the egg whites until well beaten.

2. Heat a non-stick skillet over medium heat and lightly grease it with cooking spray or olive oil.

3. Add the diced red onion to the skillet and sauté for about 2 minutes until it becomes translucent.

4. Add the chopped fresh spinach leaves to the skillet and cook for an extra 1-2 minutes, or until the spinach wilts.

5. Pour the beaten egg whites over the sautéed vegetables in the skillet.

6. Sprinkle the crumbled feta cheese evenly over the egg whites.

7. Season with iodized sea salt and black pepper.

8. Cook the omelette for 3-4 minutes, or until the edges start to set and the bottom is lightly golden.

9. Carefully flip one half of the omelette over the other half, creating a half-moon shape.

10. Cook for an extra 2-3 minutes until the inside is fully cooked, and the cheese is melted.

11. Slide the Spinach and Feta Egg White Omelette onto a plate, and enjoy your thyroid reset-friendly breakfast.

Nutritional Information (Per Serving):

- Carbs: 6 grams

- Fats: 8 grams

- Protein: 22 grams

- Sodium: 450 milligrams

SOUPS

Lemon Dill Potato Soup

Prep Time: 15 minutes
Cook Time: 30 minutes
Servings: 4

Ingredients:

- 4 cups potatoes, peeled and diced
- 1 cup onion, finely chopped
- 1/2 cup celery, finely chopped
- 1/2 cup carrots, finely chopped
- 4 cups low-sodium chicken broth
- 1/2 cup fresh dill, chopped
- 2 cloves garlic, minced
- 1/2 cup heavy cream
- 2 tablespoons unsalted butter
- 2 tablespoons all-purpose flour
- 2 tablespoons lemon juice
- Salt and pepper to taste

Instructions:

1. In a large pot, melt the butter over medium heat. Add the onions, celery, and carrots. Sauté for about 5 minutes or until the vegetables are softened.

2. Sprinkle the flour over the sautéed vegetables and stir sufficiently. Cook for an extra 2 minutes to take out the raw taste of the flour.

3. Add the diced potatoes, chicken broth, and minced garlic to the pot. Bring the mixture to a boil, then reduce the heat to low. Cover and simmer for 20 minutes, or until the potatoes are tender.

4. Using an immersion blender, carefully blend the soup until it reaches your desired level of smoothness. You can also transfer the soup to a blender in batches, but be cautious when blending hot liquids.

5. Return the blended soup to the pot, and stir in the heavy cream, lemon juice, and chopped dill. Simmer for an extra 5 minutes, allowing the flavors to meld together. Season with salt and pepper to taste.

6. Serve hot, garnished with a sprig of fresh dill if desired.

Nutritional Information (Per Serving):

- Carbs: 34g

- Fats: 14g

- Fiber: 4g

- Protein: 6g

Creamy Parsnip and Apple Soup

Prep Time: 15 minutes
Cook Time: 30 minutes
Servings: 4

Ingredients:

- 4 cups parsnips, peeled and diced

- 2 cups apples, peeled, cored, and diced

- 1 cup onion, finely chopped

- 2 cloves garlic, minced

- 4 cups low-sodium vegetable broth

- 1/2 cup heavy cream

- 2 tablespoons unsalted butter

- 2 tablespoons olive oil

- 1 teaspoon ground nutmeg

- Salt and pepper to taste

- Chopped fresh chives for garnish (optional)

Instructions:

1. In a large pot, heat the olive oil and butter over medium heat. Add the chopped onions and minced garlic. Sauté for about 5 minutes or until the onions are translucent.

2. Add the diced parsnips and apples to the pot. Keep on cooking for another 5 minutes, stirring occasionally.

3. Pour in the vegetable broth and bring the mixture to a boil. Reduce the heat to low, cover, and simmer for 20-25 minutes, or until the parsnips and apples are tender.

4. Using an immersion blender, carefully blend the soup until it's smooth and creamy. Alternatively, transfer the soup to a blender in batches, but be cautious with hot liquids.

5. Return the blended soup to the pot, and stir in the heavy cream and ground nutmeg. Simmer for an extra 5 minutes to heat through. Season with salt and pepper to taste.

6. Serve hot, garnished with chopped fresh chives if desired.

Nutritional Information (Per Serving):

- Carbs: 33g
- Fats: 18g
- Fiber: 7g
- Protein: 3g

Thai Coconut Shrimp Soup

Prep Time: 15 minutes
Cook Time: 20 minutes
Servings: 4

Ingredients:

- 1 pound large shrimp, peeled and deveined
- 2 cups coconut milk
- 4 cups low-sodium chicken broth

- 2 stalks lemongrass, cut into 3-inch pieces and smashed
- 4 slices galangal or ginger (about 1/4-inch thick)
- 4 kaffir lime leaves
- 2 tablespoons fish sauce
- 2 tablespoons lime juice
- 2 tablespoons brown sugar
- 1 red chili pepper, thinly sliced (adjust to taste)
- 1 cup button mushrooms, sliced
- 1 medium tomato, diced
- 2 cloves garlic, minced
- Fresh cilantro leaves for garnish
- Salt to taste

Instructions:

1. In a large pot, add the chicken broth, lemongrass, galangal or ginger, and kaffir lime leaves. Bring the mixture to a boil, then reduce the heat and simmer for 10 minutes to infuse the flavors.

2. While the broth simmers, heat a separate pan over medium heat. Add the shrimp and cook for 1-2 minutes on each side until they turn pink. Take out the shrimp from the pan and set them aside.

3. In the same pan, add minced garlic and sliced mushrooms. Sauté for about 3 minutes until the mushrooms begin to soften.

4. Strain the infused chicken broth into the pot to take out the lemongrass, galangal or ginger, and kaffir lime leaves.

5. Stir in the coconut milk, fish sauce, lime juice, brown sugar, and sliced red chili pepper. Simmer for another 5 minutes, allowing the flavors to meld together.

6. Add the diced tomatoes and cooked shrimp to the soup. Simmer for an extra 2-3 minutes until the shrimp are heated through.

7. Season the soup with salt to taste.

8. Serve hot, garnished with fresh cilantro leaves.

Nutritional Information (Per Serving):

- Carbs: 17g

- Fats: 30g

- Fiber: 2g

- Protein: 21g

White Bean and Kale Soup

Prep Time: 15 minutes
Cook Time: 30 minutes
Servings: 4

Ingredients:

- 2 cups dried white beans, soaked overnight and drained

- 1 cup onion, finely chopped

- 1 cup carrots, diced

- 1 cup celery, diced

- 2 cloves garlic, minced

- 6 cups low-sodium chicken or vegetable broth

- 4 cups kale, stems removed and chopped

- 2 bay leaves

- 1 teaspoon dried thyme

- 2 tablespoons olive oil

- Salt and pepper to taste

- Grated Parmesan cheese for garnish (optional)

Instructions:

1. In a large pot, heat the olive oil over medium heat. Add the chopped onions, diced carrots, and diced celery. Sauté for about 5 minutes, or until the vegetables begin to soften.

2. Add the minced garlic to the pot and sauté for an extra minute, until fragrant.

3. Add the soaked and drained white beans, chicken or vegetable broth, bay leaves, and dried thyme to the pot. Bring the mixture to a boil, then reduce the heat to low. Cover and simmer for 20-25 minutes, or until the white beans are tender.

4. Stir in the chopped kale and continue to simmer for an extra 5 minutes, or until the kale is wilted and tender.

5. Take out the bay leaves from the soup and discard them.

6. Season the soup with salt and pepper to taste.

7. Serve hot, garnished with grated Parmesan cheese if desired.

Nutritional Information (Per Serving):

- Carbs: 35g

- Fats: 6g

- Fiber: 6g

- Protein: 14g

Creamy Spinach and Artichoke Soup

Prep Time: 15 minutes
Cook Time: 25 minutes
Servings: 4

Ingredients:

- 2 cups fresh spinach, chopped

- 1 cup canned artichoke hearts, drained and chopped

- 1 cup onion, finely chopped

- 2 cloves garlic, minced

- 4 cups low-sodium vegetable broth

- 1 cup heavy cream

- 1/2 cup grated Parmesan cheese

- 2 tablespoons unsalted butter

- 2 tablespoons olive oil

- 2 tablespoons all-purpose flour

- 1/2 teaspoon dried thyme
- Salt and pepper to taste
- Grated Parmesan cheese and fresh chopped parsley for garnish (optional)

Instructions:

1. In a large pot, heat the olive oil and butter over medium heat. Add the chopped onions and minced garlic. Sauté for about 5 minutes, or until the onions are translucent.

2. Sprinkle the all-purpose flour over the sautéed onions and garlic. Stir sufficiently and cook for an extra 2 minutes to take out the raw taste of the flour.

3. Slowly pour in the vegetable broth while continuously stirring to avoid lumps. Bring the mixture to a simmer.

4. Stir in the chopped spinach, chopped artichoke hearts, and dried thyme. Simmer for 10-15 minutes, or until the spinach is wilted and tender.

5. Reduce the heat to low, and stir in the heavy cream and grated Parmesan cheese. Cook for an extra 5 minutes, stirring occasionally, until the soup is heated through and the cheese is melted.

6. Season the soup with salt and pepper to taste.

7. Serve hot, garnished with additional grated Parmesan cheese and fresh chopped parsley if desired.

Nutritional Information (Per Serving):

- Carbs: 12g
- Fats: 31g
- Fiber: 2g
- Protein: 7g

Cucumber Gazpacho

Prep Time: 15 minutes
Cook Time: 0 minutes (no cooking required)
Servings: 4

Ingredients:

- 4 cups cucumber, peeled, seeded, and diced
- 2 cups ripe tomatoes, diced
- 1/2 cup red bell pepper, diced
- 1/2 cup red onion, finely chopped
- 2 cloves garlic, minced
- 2 cups low-sodium vegetable broth
- 1/4 cup fresh basil leaves, chopped
- 1/4 cup fresh cilantro leaves, chopped
- 2 tablespoons red wine vinegar
- 2 tablespoons olive oil
- 1 teaspoon salt
- 1/2 teaspoon black pepper
- Greek yogurt or sour cream for garnish (optional)

Instructions:

1. In a blender or food processor, add the diced cucumbers, diced tomatoes, diced red bell pepper, finely chopped red onion, and minced garlic.

2. Pulse the mixture until it reaches your desired level of smoothness. If you prefer a chunkier texture, pulse a few times. For a smoother consistency, blend until fully smooth.

3. Transfer the blended mixture to a large bowl.

4. Stir in the low-sodium vegetable broth, chopped fresh basil leaves, chopped fresh cilantro leaves, red wine vinegar, olive oil, salt, and black pepper. Mix sufficiently to combine.

5. Refrigerate the gazpacho for at least 1 hour before serving to allow the flavors to meld.

6. Serve cold, garnished with a dollop of Greek yogurt or sour cream if desired.

Nutritional Information (Per Serving):

- Carbs: 10g

- Fats: 7g

- Fiber: 2g

- Protein: 2g

Roasted Garlic and Potato Soup

Prep Time: 15 minutes
Cook Time: 50 minutes
Servings: 4

Ingredients:

- 4 cups potatoes, peeled and diced

- 1 cup onion, finely chopped

- 1/4 cup roasted garlic cloves (about 1 head of garlic)

- 4 cups low-sodium vegetable broth

- 1 cup heavy cream

- 2 tablespoons unsalted butter

- 2 tablespoons olive oil

- 1 teaspoon dried thyme

- Salt and pepper to taste

- Chopped fresh chives for garnish (optional)

Instructions:

1. Turn on your oven and set it to 400°F (200°C) to preheat.

2. Cut the top off the head of garlic to expose the cloves. Place the garlic head on a piece of aluminum foil, drizzle with a bit of olive oil, and wrap it tightly in the foil. Roast the garlic in the preheated oven for 30-35 minutes, or until the cloves are soft and golden. Once done, take out the cloves from their skins.

3. In a large pot, heat the olive oil and butter over medium heat. Add the chopped onions and sauté for about 5 minutes until they become translucent.

4. Add the diced potatoes to the pot and keep on cooking for another 5 minutes, stirring occasionally.

5. Pour in the low-sodium vegetable broth, add the roasted garlic cloves, and sprinkle in the dried thyme. Bring the mixture to a boil, then reduce the heat to low. Cover and simmer for 20-25 minutes, or until the potatoes are tender.

6. Using an immersion blender, carefully blend the soup until it reaches your desired level of smoothness. Alternatively, transfer the soup to a blender in batches, but be cautious when blending hot liquids.

7. Return the blended soup to the pot, and stir in the heavy cream. Simmer for an extra 5 minutes to heat through.

8. Season the soup with salt and pepper to taste.

9. Serve hot, garnished with chopped fresh chives if desired.

Nutritional Information (Per Serving):

- Carbs: 29g
- Fats: 21g
- Fiber: 2g
- Protein: 4g

Moroccan Lentil Soup

Prep Time: 15 minutes
Cook Time: 40 minutes
Servings: 4

Ingredients:

- 1 cup dried red lentils
- 1 cup onion, finely chopped
- 1/2 cup carrots, diced
- 1/2 cup celery, diced

- 2 cloves garlic, minced
- 4 cups low-sodium vegetable broth
- 1 cup canned diced tomatoes
- 2 tablespoons olive oil
- 1 tablespoon ground cumin
- 1 teaspoon ground coriander
- 1/2 teaspoon ground turmeric
- 1/2 teaspoon paprika
- 1/4 teaspoon ground cinnamon
- Salt and pepper to taste
- Fresh cilantro leaves for garnish (optional)
- Lemon wedges for serving (optional)

Instructions:

1. In a large pot, heat the olive oil over medium heat. Add the chopped onions, diced carrots, and diced celery. Sauté for about 5 minutes until the vegetables soften.

2. Add the minced garlic to the pot and sauté for an extra minute until fragrant.

3. Rinse the red lentils thoroughly under cold water, then add them to the pot along with the ground cumin, ground coriander, ground turmeric, paprika, and ground cinnamon. Stir sufficiently to coat the lentils and vegetables with the spices.

4. Pour in the low-sodium vegetable broth and diced tomatoes. Bring the mixture to a boil, then reduce the heat to low. Cover and simmer for 30 minutes, or until the lentils are tender.

5. Use an immersion blender to carefully blend the soup until it reaches your desired level of smoothness. Alternatively, transfer the soup to a blender in batches, but be cautious when blending hot liquids.

6. Season the soup with salt and pepper to taste.

7. Serve hot, garnished with fresh cilantro leaves and lemon wedges if desired.

Nutritional Information (Per Serving):

- Carbs: 32g

- Fats: 7g

- Fiber: 4g

- Protein: 10g

Creamy Tomato and Red Pepper Soup

Prep Time: 15 minutes
Cook Time: 35 minutes
Servings: 4

Ingredients:

- 4 cups canned crushed tomatoes

- 2 cups roasted red bell peppers, diced

- 1 cup onion, finely chopped

- 2 cloves garlic, minced

- 2 cups low-sodium vegetable broth

- 1 cup heavy cream

- 2 tablespoons unsalted butter

- 2 tablespoons olive oil

- 1 teaspoon dried basil

- 1/2 teaspoon dried oregano

- 1/4 teaspoon red pepper flakes (adjust to taste)

- Salt and pepper to taste

- Fresh basil leaves for garnish (optional)

Instructions:

1. In a large pot, heat the olive oil and butter over medium heat. Add the chopped onions and sauté for about 5 minutes until they become translucent.

2. Add the minced garlic to the pot and sauté for an extra minute until fragrant.

3. Stir in the diced roasted red bell peppers and keep on cooking for another 5 minutes.

4. Pour in the canned crushed tomatoes, low-sodium vegetable broth, dried basil, dried oregano, and red pepper flakes. Mix sufficiently to combine.

5. Bring the mixture to a boil, then reduce the heat to low. Cover and simmer for 20-25 minutes, allowing the flavors to meld.

6. Use an immersion blender to carefully blend the soup until it's smooth and creamy. Alternatively, transfer the soup to a blender in batches, but be cautious when blending hot liquids.

7. Return the blended soup to the pot and stir in the heavy cream. Simmer for an extra 5 minutes to heat through.

8. Season the soup with salt and pepper to taste.

9. Serve hot, garnished with fresh basil leaves if desired.

Nutritional Information (Per Serving):

- Carbs: 18g
- Fats: 26g
- Fiber: 4g
- Protein: 4g

Chicken and Rice Congee

Prep Time: 10 minutes
Cook Time: 1 hour
Servings: 4

Ingredients:

- 1 cup white rice
- 4 cups low-sodium chicken broth
- 2 cups water
- 1 cup cooked chicken breast, shredded
- 1/4 cup green onions, thinly sliced
- 1 tablespoon fresh ginger, minced
- 1 tablespoon vegetable oil
- 1/2 teaspoon salt (adjust to taste)
- 1/4 teaspoon white pepper (adjust to taste)
- Soy sauce for serving (optional)
- Sesame oil for serving (optional)

Instructions:

1. Rinse the white rice thoroughly under cold water and drain.

2. In a large pot, heat the vegetable oil over medium heat. Add the minced ginger and sliced green onions. Sauté for about 2 minutes until fragrant.

3. Add the rinsed rice to the pot and keep on cooking for another 2 minutes, stirring occasionally.

4. Pour in the low-sodium chicken broth and water. Bring the mixture to a boil.

5. Reduce the heat to low, cover the pot, and simmer for about 45-50 minutes, stirring occasionally, until the rice has broken down and the congee has thickened to your desired consistency.

6. Stir in the shredded cooked chicken breast and continue to simmer for an extra 5-10 minutes until the chicken is heated through.

7. Season the congee with salt and white pepper to taste.

8. Serve hot, optionally garnished with additional sliced green onions. Offer soy sauce and sesame oil as condiments at the table for drizzling on top if desired.

Nutritional Information (Per Serving):

- Carbs: 38g

- Fats: 4g

- Fiber: 1g

- Protein: 17g

Creamy Carrot Soup

Prep Time: 15 minutes
Cook Time: 30 minutes
Servings: 4

Ingredients:

- 4 cups carrots, peeled and sliced

- 1 cup onion, finely chopped

- 2 cloves garlic, minced

- 4 cups low-sodium vegetable broth

- 1 cup heavy cream

- 2 tablespoons unsalted butter

- 2 tablespoons olive oil

- 1/2 teaspoon ground cumin

- 1/2 teaspoon ground coriander

- 1/4 teaspoon ground nutmeg

- Salt and pepper to taste

- Fresh parsley leaves for garnish (optional)

Instructions:

1. In a large pot, heat the olive oil and butter over medium heat. Add the chopped onions and sauté for about 5 minutes until they become translucent.

2. Add the minced garlic to the pot and sauté for an extra minute until fragrant.

3. Stir in the sliced carrots and keep on cooking for another 5 minutes.

4. Pour in the low-sodium vegetable broth, ground cumin, ground coriander, and ground nutmeg. Mix sufficiently to combine.

5. Bring the mixture to a boil, then reduce the heat to low. Cover and simmer for 20-25 minutes, or until the carrots are tender.

6. Use an immersion blender to carefully blend the soup until it reaches your desired level of smoothness. Alternatively, transfer the soup to a blender in batches, but be cautious when blending hot liquids.

7. Return the blended soup to the pot and stir in the heavy cream. Simmer for an extra 5 minutes to heat through.

8. Season the soup with salt and pepper to taste.

9. Serve hot, garnished with fresh parsley leaves if desired.

Nutritional Information (Per Serving):

- Carbs: 17g

- Fats: 21g

- Fiber: 3g

- Protein: 4g

Potato Leek Soup

Prep Time: 15 minutes
Cook Time: 40 minutes
Servings: 4

Ingredients:

- 4 cups potatoes, peeled and diced

- 2 cups leeks, white and light green parts, thinly sliced

- 1 cup onion, finely chopped

- 2 cloves garlic, minced

- 4 cups low-sodium vegetable broth

- 1 cup heavy cream

- 2 tablespoons unsalted butter
- 2 tablespoons olive oil
- 1/2 teaspoon dried thyme
- Salt and pepper to taste
- Fresh chives for garnish (optional)

Instructions:

1. In a large pot, heat the olive oil and butter over medium heat. Add the chopped onions and thinly sliced leeks. Sauté for about 5 minutes until they become soft and translucent.

2. Add the minced garlic to the pot and sauté for an extra minute until fragrant.

3. Stir in the diced potatoes and dried thyme. Keep on cooking for another 5 minutes, stirring occasionally.

4. Pour in the low-sodium vegetable broth. Bring the mixture to a boil, then reduce the heat to low. Cover and simmer for 20-25 minutes, or until the potatoes are tender.

5. Use an immersion blender to carefully blend the soup until it reaches your desired level of smoothness. Alternatively, transfer the soup to a blender in batches, but be cautious when blending hot liquids.

6. Return the blended soup to the pot and stir in the heavy cream. Simmer for an extra 5 minutes to heat through.

7. Season the soup with salt and pepper to taste.

8. Serve hot, garnished with fresh chives if desired.

Nutritional Information (Per Serving):

- Carbs: 30g
- Fats: 23g
- Fiber: 3g
- Protein: 4g

Butternut Squash Bisque

Prep Time: 15 minutes
Cook Time: 45 minutes
Servings: 4

Ingredients:

- 4 cups butternut squash, peeled and diced
- 1 cup onion, finely chopped
- 2 cloves garlic, minced
- 4 cups low-sodium vegetable broth
- 1 cup heavy cream
- 2 tablespoons unsalted butter
- 2 tablespoons olive oil
- 1/2 teaspoon ground cinnamon
- 1/4 teaspoon ground nutmeg
- Salt and pepper to taste
- Fresh thyme leaves for garnish (optional)

Instructions:

1. In a large pot, heat the olive oil and butter over medium heat. Add the chopped onions and sauté for about 5 minutes until they become soft and translucent.

2. Add the minced garlic to the pot and sauté for an extra minute until fragrant.

3. Stir in the diced butternut squash, ground cinnamon, and ground nutmeg. Keep on cooking for another 5 minutes, stirring occasionally.

4. Pour in the low-sodium vegetable broth. Bring the mixture to a boil, then reduce the heat to low. Cover and simmer for 30-35 minutes, or until the butternut squash is tender.

5. Use an immersion blender to carefully blend the soup until it reaches your desired level of smoothness. Alternatively, transfer the soup to a blender in batches, but be cautious when blending hot liquids.

6. Return the blended soup to the pot and stir in the heavy cream. Simmer for an extra 5 minutes to heat through.

7. Season the soup with salt and pepper to taste.

8. Serve hot, garnished with fresh thyme leaves if desired.

Nutritional Information (Per Serving):

- Carbs: 24g

- Fats: 23g

- Fiber: 3g

- Protein: 4g

Tomato Basil Soup

Prep Time: 15 minutes
Cook Time: 30 minutes
Servings: 4

Ingredients:

- 4 cups canned crushed tomatoes

- 1 cup onion, finely chopped

- 2 cloves garlic, minced

- 4 cups low-sodium vegetable broth

- 1 cup heavy cream

- 2 tablespoons unsalted butter

- 2 tablespoons olive oil

- 1/4 cup fresh basil leaves, chopped

- 1/4 cup fresh parsley leaves, chopped

- Salt and pepper to taste

- Grated Parmesan cheese for garnish (optional)

Instructions:

1. In a large pot, heat the olive oil and butter over medium heat. Add the chopped onions and sauté for about 5 minutes until they become soft and translucent.

2. Add the minced garlic to the pot and sauté for an extra minute until fragrant.

3. Pour in the canned crushed tomatoes and low-sodium vegetable broth. Mix sufficiently to combine.

4. Bring the mixture to a boil, then reduce the heat to low. Cover and simmer for 20-25 minutes, allowing the flavors to meld.

5. Stir in the chopped fresh basil leaves and chopped fresh parsley leaves. Simmer for an extra 5 minutes.

6. Use an immersion blender to carefully blend the soup until it reaches your desired level of smoothness. Alternatively, transfer the soup to a blender in batches, but be cautious when blending hot liquids.

7. Return the blended soup to the pot and stir in the heavy cream. Simmer for an extra 5 minutes to heat through.

8. Season the soup with salt and pepper to taste.

9. Serve hot, garnished with grated Parmesan cheese if desired.

Nutritional Information (Per Serving):

- Carbs: 21g

- Fats: 27g

- Fiber: 3g

- Protein: 5g

Creamy Mushroom Soup

Prep Time: 15 minutes
Cook Time: 35 minutes
Servings: 4

Ingredients:

- 4 cups fresh mushrooms, sliced

- 1 cup onion, finely chopped

- 2 cloves garlic, minced
- 4 cups low-sodium vegetable broth
- 1 cup heavy cream
- 2 tablespoons unsalted butter
- 2 tablespoons olive oil
- 1/4 cup all-purpose flour
- 1/2 teaspoon dried thyme
- Salt and pepper to taste
- Fresh parsley leaves for garnish (optional)

Instructions:

1. In a large pot, heat the olive oil and butter over medium heat. Add the chopped onions and sauté for about 5 minutes until they become soft and translucent.

2. Add the minced garlic to the pot and sauté for an extra minute until fragrant.

3. Stir in the sliced mushrooms and dried thyme. Keep on cooking for about 10 minutes, or until the mushrooms have released their moisture and become tender.

4. Sprinkle the all-purpose flour over the mushroom mixture. Stir sufficiently and cook for an extra 2 minutes to take out the raw taste of the flour.

5. Pour in the low-sodium vegetable broth while continuously stirring to avoid lumps. Bring the mixture to a simmer.

6. Reduce the heat to low, cover, and simmer for 10-15 minutes, allowing the flavors to meld.

7. Use an immersion blender to carefully blend the soup until it reaches your desired level of smoothness. Alternatively, transfer the soup to a blender in batches, but be cautious when blending hot liquids.

8. Return the blended soup to the pot and stir in the heavy cream. Simmer for an extra 5 minutes to heat through.

9. Season the soup with salt and pepper to taste.

10. Serve hot, garnished with fresh parsley leaves if desired.

Nutritional Information (Per Serving):

- Carbs: 15g
- Fats: 28g
- Fiber: 2g
- Protein: 4g

Chicken and Rice Soup

Prep Time: 15 minutes
Cook Time: 40 minutes
Servings: 4

Ingredients:

- 1 cup cooked chicken breast, shredded
- 1 cup white rice
- 1 cup carrots, diced
- 1/2 cup celery, diced
- 1/2 cup onion, finely chopped
- 2 cloves garlic, minced
- 4 cups low-sodium chicken broth
- 2 tablespoons olive oil
- 1/2 teaspoon dried thyme
- Salt and pepper to taste
- Fresh parsley leaves for garnish (optional)

Instructions:

1. In a large pot, heat the olive oil over medium heat. Add the chopped onions and sauté for about 5 minutes until they become soft and translucent.

2. Add the minced garlic to the pot and sauté for an extra minute until fragrant.

3. Stir in the diced carrots and diced celery. Keep on cooking for another 5 minutes.

4. Pour in the white rice and dried thyme. Cook for an extra 2 minutes, stirring occasionally.

5. Add the low-sodium chicken broth to the pot. Bring the mixture to a boil.

6. Reduce the heat to low, cover, and simmer for 15-20 minutes, or until the rice and vegetables are tender.

7. Stir in the shredded cooked chicken breast and simmer for an extra 5 minutes to heat through.

8. Season the soup with salt and pepper to taste.

9. Serve hot, optionally garnished with fresh parsley leaves.

Nutritional Information (Per Serving):

- Carbs: 28g

- Fats: 9g

- Fiber: 2g

- Protein: 20g

Roasted Red Pepper and Tomato Soup

Prep Time: 15 minutes
Cook Time: 40 minutes
Servings: 4

Ingredients:

- 4 cups canned crushed tomatoes

- 2 cups roasted red bell peppers, diced

- 1 cup onion, finely chopped

- 2 cloves garlic, minced

- 4 cups low-sodium vegetable broth

- 1 cup heavy cream

- 2 tablespoons unsalted butter

- 2 tablespoons olive oil
- 1 teaspoon dried basil
- 1/2 teaspoon dried oregano
- Salt and pepper to taste
- Fresh basil leaves for garnish (optional)

Instructions:

1. In a large pot, heat the olive oil and butter over medium heat. Add the chopped onions and sauté for about 5 minutes until they become soft and translucent.

2. Add the minced garlic to the pot and sauté for an extra minute until fragrant.

3. Stir in the diced roasted red bell peppers and keep on cooking for another 5 minutes.

4. Pour in the canned crushed tomatoes, dried basil, dried oregano, and low-sodium vegetable broth. Mix sufficiently to combine.

5. Bring the mixture to a boil, then reduce the heat to low. Cover and simmer for 20-25 minutes, allowing the flavors to meld.

6. Use an immersion blender to carefully blend the soup until it's smooth and creamy. Alternatively, transfer the soup to a blender in batches, but be cautious when blending hot liquids.

7. Return the blended soup to the pot and stir in the heavy cream. Simmer for an extra 5 minutes to heat through.

8. Season the soup with salt and pepper to taste.

9. Serve hot, garnished with fresh basil leaves if desired.

Nutritional Information (Per Serving):

- Carbs: 21g
- Fats: 27g
- Fiber: 3g
- Protein: 4g

Broccoli Cheddar Soup

Prep Time: 15 minutes
Cook Time: 30 minutes
Servings: 4

Ingredients:

- 4 cups fresh broccoli florets, chopped
- 1 cup onion, finely chopped
- 2 cloves garlic, minced
- 4 cups low-sodium vegetable broth
- 1 cup heavy cream
- 2 cups shredded cheddar cheese
- 2 tablespoons unsalted butter
- 2 tablespoons olive oil
- 1/4 cup all-purpose flour
- 1/4 teaspoon nutmeg
- Salt and pepper to taste
- Fresh chives for garnish (optional)

Instructions:

1. In a large pot, heat the olive oil and butter over medium heat. Add the chopped onions and sauté for about 5 minutes until they become soft and translucent.

2. Add the minced garlic to the pot and sauté for an extra minute until fragrant.

3. Stir in the chopped fresh broccoli florets. Keep on cooking for another 5 minutes.

4. Sprinkle the all-purpose flour over the broccoli mixture. Stir sufficiently and cook for an extra 2 minutes, stirring occasionally to take out the raw taste of the flour.

5. Pour in the low-sodium vegetable broth while continuously stirring to avoid lumps. Bring the mixture to a simmer.

6. Reduce the heat to low, cover, and simmer for 15-20 minutes, or until the broccoli is tender.

7. Use an immersion blender to carefully blend the soup until it reaches your desired level of smoothness. Alternatively, transfer the soup to a blender in batches, but be cautious when blending hot liquids.

8. Return the blended soup to the pot and stir in the heavy cream and shredded cheddar cheese. Simmer for an extra 5 minutes to heat through and melt the cheese.

9. Season the soup with nutmeg, salt, and pepper to taste.

10. Serve hot, optionally garnished with fresh chives.

Nutritional Information (Per Serving):

- Carbs: 19g
- Fats: 47g
- Fiber: 3g
- Protein: 18g

Creamy Cauliflower Soup

Prep Time: 15 minutes
Cook Time: 30 minutes
Servings: 4

Ingredients:

- 1 large head of cauliflower, chopped into florets
- 1 cup onion, finely chopped
- 2 cloves garlic, minced
- 4 cups low-sodium vegetable broth
- 1 cup heavy cream
- 2 tablespoons unsalted butter
- 2 tablespoons olive oil
- 1/2 teaspoon ground cumin

- 1/4 teaspoon ground nutmeg
- Salt and pepper to taste
- Fresh parsley leaves for garnish (optional)

Instructions:

1. In a large pot, heat the olive oil and butter over medium heat. Add the chopped onions and sauté for about 5 minutes until they become soft and translucent.

2. Add the minced garlic to the pot and sauté for an extra minute until fragrant.

3. Stir in the chopped cauliflower florets. Keep on cooking for another 5 minutes.

4. Pour in the low-sodium vegetable broth, ground cumin, and ground nutmeg. Mix sufficiently to combine.

5. Bring the mixture to a boil, then reduce the heat to low. Cover and simmer for 20-25 minutes, or until the cauliflower is tender.

6. Use an immersion blender to carefully blend the soup until it reaches your desired level of smoothness. Alternatively, transfer the soup to a blender in batches, but be cautious when blending hot liquids.

7. Return the blended soup to the pot and stir in the heavy cream. Simmer for an extra 5 minutes to heat through.

8. Season the soup with salt and pepper to taste.

9. Serve hot, optionally garnished with fresh parsley leaves.

Nutritional Information (Per Serving):

- Carbs: 17g
- Fats: 26g
- Fiber: 4g
- Protein: 5g

Coconut Curry Lentil Soup

Prep Time: 15 minutes
Cook Time: 40 minutes
Servings: 4

Ingredients:

- 1 cup dried red lentils
- 1 cup onion, finely chopped
- 2 cloves garlic, minced
- 4 cups low-sodium vegetable broth
- 1 cup canned coconut milk
- 2 tablespoons olive oil
- 2 tablespoons curry powder
- 1 teaspoon ground turmeric
- 1/2 teaspoon ground cumin
- 1/4 teaspoon cayenne pepper (adjust to taste)
- Salt and pepper to taste
- Fresh cilantro leaves for garnish (optional)

Instructions:

1. In a large pot, heat the olive oil over medium heat. Add the chopped onions and sauté for about 5 minutes until they become soft and translucent.

2. Add the minced garlic to the pot and sauté for an extra minute until fragrant.

3. Stir in the curry powder, ground turmeric, ground cumin, and cayenne pepper. Cook for another 2 minutes, stirring constantly to toast the spices.

4. Add the dried red lentils to the pot and pour in the low-sodium vegetable broth. Mix sufficiently to combine.

5. Bring the mixture to a boil, then reduce the heat to low. Cover and simmer for 20-25 minutes, or until the lentils are tender and properly cooked.

6. Stir in the canned coconut milk and simmer for an extra 5 minutes to heat through.

7. Season the soup with salt and pepper to taste.

8. Serve hot, optionally garnished with fresh cilantro leaves.

Nutritional Information (Per Serving):

- Carbs: 35g
- Fats: 18g
- Fiber: 10g
- Protein: 13g

SALADS

Radicchio and Orange Salad

Prep Time: 15 minutes
Cook Time: 0 minutes
Number of Servings: 4

Ingredients:

- 1 large head of radicchio, chopped
- 2 large oranges, peeled and segmented
- 1/2 cup red onion, thinly sliced
- 1/4 cup toasted pine nuts
- 1/4 cup crumbled feta cheese
- 2 tablespoons fresh parsley, chopped

For the Dressing:

- 2 tablespoons extra-virgin olive oil
- 1 tablespoon red wine vinegar
- 1 tablespoon honey
- Salt and freshly ground black pepper, to taste

Instructions:

1. In a large salad bowl, add the chopped radicchio, orange segments, thinly sliced red onion, and toasted pine nuts.

2. In a separate small bowl, whisk the olive oil, red wine vinegar, honey, salt, and freshly ground black pepper to make the dressing.

3. Drizzle the dressing over the salad ingredients and toss gently to coat.

4. Sprinkle the crumbled feta cheese and chopped fresh parsley over the top of the salad.

5. Serve immediately as a refreshing side dish or light main course.

Nutritional Information (per serving):

- Carbs: 18g

- Fats: 12g

- Fiber: 3g

- Protein: 4g

Roasted Eggplant and Tomato Salad
Prep Time: 15 minutes
Cook Time: 25 minutes
Number of Servings: 4

Ingredients:

- 2 medium eggplants, diced into 1-inch cubes

- 2 cups cherry tomatoes, halved

- 1/2 cup red onion, thinly sliced

- 3 cloves garlic, minced

- 2 tablespoons olive oil

- 1 teaspoon dried oregano

- 1/2 teaspoon salt

- 1/4 teaspoon black pepper

- 2 tablespoons fresh basil leaves, chopped

- 1/4 cup crumbled goat cheese (optional)

Instructions:

1. Turn on your oven and set it to 425°F (220°C) to preheat.

2. In a large mixing bowl, add the diced eggplants, halved cherry tomatoes, thinly sliced red onion, minced garlic, olive oil, dried oregano, salt, and black pepper. Toss to coat the vegetables evenly.

3. Spread the vegetable mixture in a single layer on a baking sheet lined with parchment paper.

4. Roast the vegetables in the preheated oven for 20-25 minutes or until the eggplants are tender and slightly browned, stirring once halfway through the cooking time.

5. Take out the roasted vegetables from the oven and let them cool slightly.

6. Transfer the roasted eggplant and tomato mixture to a serving platter.

7. Sprinkle the chopped fresh basil leaves over the top.

8. If desired, crumble the goat cheese over the salad.

9. Serve the roasted eggplant and tomato salad warm or at room temperature.

Nutritional Information (per serving):

- Carbs: 19g

- Fats: 7g

- Fiber: 5g

- Protein: 4g

Tuna and Avocado Salad
Prep Time: 10 minutes
Cook Time: 0 minutes
Number of Servings: 2

Ingredients:

- 2 (5-ounce) cans of tuna in water, drained

- 1 large avocado, diced

- 1/4 cup red onion, finely chopped

- 1/4 cup celery, diced

- 2 tablespoons mayonnaise

- 1 tablespoon lemon juice

- 1/2 teaspoon Dijon mustard

- Salt and freshly ground black pepper, to taste

- Fresh parsley leaves for garnish (optional)

Instructions:

1. In a mixing bowl, add the drained tuna, diced avocado, finely chopped red onion, and diced celery.

2. In a separate small bowl, whisk the mayonnaise, lemon juice, Dijon mustard, salt, and freshly ground black pepper to make the dressing.

3. Drizzle the dressing over the tuna and avocado mixture.

4. Gently toss the ingredients together until everything is well coated with the dressing.

5. Divide the tuna and avocado salad into two serving plates.

6. If desired, garnish with fresh parsley leaves.

7. Serve immediately as a delicious and satisfying salad.

Nutritional Information (per serving):

- Carbs: 8g
- Fats: 27g
- Fiber: 5g
- Protein: 27g

Jicama and Mango Salad
Prep Time: 20 minutes
Cook Time: 0 minutes
Number of Servings: 4

Ingredients:

- 1 medium jicama, peeled and julienned
- 2 ripe mangoes, peeled, pitted, and diced
- 1/2 cup red bell pepper, diced
- 1/4 cup red onion, finely chopped
- 1/4 cup fresh cilantro leaves, chopped
- Juice of 2 limes
- 1 tablespoon honey

- 1/2 teaspoon ground cumin

- 1/4 teaspoon chili powder

- Salt and freshly ground black pepper, to taste

Instructions:

1. In a large mixing bowl, add the julienned jicama, diced mangoes, diced red bell pepper, finely chopped red onion, and chopped fresh cilantro leaves.

2. In a separate small bowl, whisk the lime juice, honey, ground cumin, chili powder, salt, and freshly ground black pepper to make the dressing.

3. Drizzle the dressing over the jicama and mango mixture.

4. Gently toss the ingredients together until well coated with the dressing.

5. Divide the jicama and mango salad into four serving plates.

6. Serve immediately as a refreshing and flavorful salad.

Nutritional Information (per serving):

- Carbs: 34g

- Fats: 1g

- Fiber: 7g

- Protein: 2g

Red Cabbage Slaw with Lemon Dressing

Prep Time: 15 minutes
Cook Time: 0 minutes
Number of Servings: 4

Ingredients:

For the Slaw:

- 4 cups red cabbage, thinly sliced

- 1 large carrot, grated

- 1/2 red bell pepper, thinly sliced

- 1/4 cup red onion, finely chopped
- 2 tablespoons fresh parsley leaves, chopped

For the Lemon Dressing:

- Juice of 2 lemons
- 2 tablespoons extra-virgin olive oil
- 1 teaspoon honey
- 1/2 teaspoon Dijon mustard
- Salt and freshly ground black pepper, to taste

Instructions:

1. In a large mixing bowl, add the thinly sliced red cabbage, grated carrot, thinly sliced red bell pepper, finely chopped red onion, and chopped fresh parsley leaves.

2. In a separate small bowl, whisk the lemon juice, extra-virgin olive oil, honey, Dijon mustard, salt, and freshly ground black pepper to make the dressing.

3. Drizzle the lemon dressing over the slaw ingredients.

4. Gently toss the slaw to ensure it's well coated with the dressing.

5. Divide the red cabbage slaw into four serving plates.

6. Serve immediately as a zesty and crunchy salad.

Nutritional Information (per serving):

- Carbs: 12g
- Fats: 7g
- Fiber: 3g
- Protein: 2g

Spinach and Strawberry Salad

Prep Time: 15 minutes
Cook Time: 0 minutes
Number of Servings: 4

Ingredients:

- 8 cups fresh spinach leaves, washed and dried
- 2 cups fresh strawberries, hulled and sliced
- 1/2 cup red onion, thinly sliced
- 1/4 cup slivered almonds, toasted
- 1/4 cup crumbled feta cheese

For the Dressing:

- 3 tablespoons balsamic vinegar
- 2 tablespoons extra-virgin olive oil
- 1 tablespoon honey
- 1/2 teaspoon Dijon mustard
- Salt and freshly ground black pepper, to taste

Instructions:

1. In a large salad bowl, place the fresh spinach leaves.
2. Top the spinach with the sliced fresh strawberries, thinly sliced red onion, toasted slivered almonds, and crumbled feta cheese.
3. In a separate small bowl, whisk the balsamic vinegar, extra-virgin olive oil, honey, Dijon mustard, salt, and freshly ground black pepper to make the dressing.
4. Drizzle the dressing over the salad ingredients.
5. Gently toss the salad to ensure everything is well coated with the dressing.
6. Divide the spinach and strawberry salad into four serving plates.
7. Serve immediately as a delightful and nutritious salad.

Nutritional Information (per serving):

- Carbs: 16g
- Fats: 13g
- Fiber: 4g
- Protein: 5g

Roasted Butternut Squash Salad

Prep Time: 15 minutes
Cook Time: 25 minutes
Number of Servings: 4

Ingredients:

For the Salad:

- 4 cups butternut squash, peeled, seeded, and diced into 1-inch cubes
- 2 tablespoons olive oil
- Salt and freshly ground black pepper, to taste
- 8 cups mixed greens (such as spinach and arugula)

For the Dressing:

- 3 tablespoons balsamic vinegar
- 2 tablespoons extra-virgin olive oil
- 1 tablespoon honey
- 1/2 teaspoon Dijon mustard
- 1/4 cup toasted pumpkin seeds
- 1/4 cup crumbled goat cheese (optional)

Instructions:

1. Turn on your oven and set it to 425°F (220°C) to preheat.

2. In a large mixing bowl, toss the diced butternut squash with olive oil, salt, and freshly ground black pepper.

3. Spread the seasoned butternut squash in a single layer on a baking sheet.

4. Roast in the preheated oven for 20-25 minutes, or until the squash is tender and slightly caramelized, flipping them halfway through the cooking time.

5. While the butternut squash is roasting, prepare the dressing. In a small bowl, whisk the balsamic vinegar, extra-virgin olive oil, honey, Dijon mustard, and a pinch of salt and pepper.

6. Once the butternut squash is done roasting, remove it from the oven and let it cool slightly.

7. In a large salad bowl, add the mixed greens and the roasted butternut squash.

8. Drizzle the dressing over the salad and toss gently to coat.

9. Sprinkle toasted pumpkin seeds and crumbled goat cheese (if using) over the top of the salad.

10. Serve immediately as a warm and savory salad.

Nutritional Information (per serving):

- Carbs: 23g

- Fats: 20g

- Fiber: 5g

- Protein: 4g

Broccoli and Apple Salad
Prep Time: 15 minutes
Cook Time: 0 minutes
Number of Servings: 4

Ingredients:

- 4 cups broccoli florets, blanched and cooled

- 2 medium apples, cored and diced

- 1/2 cup red onion, finely chopped

- 1/4 cup raisins

- 1/4 cup mayonnaise

- 2 tablespoons Greek yogurt

- 2 tablespoons apple cider vinegar

- 1 tablespoon honey

- 1/4 teaspoon celery seed

- Salt and freshly ground black pepper, to taste

- 1/4 cup chopped pecans (optional)

Instructions:

1. In a large mixing bowl, add the blanched and cooled broccoli florets, diced apples, finely chopped red onion, and raisins.

2. In a separate small bowl, whisk the mayonnaise, Greek yogurt, apple cider vinegar, honey, celery seed, salt, and freshly ground black pepper to make the dressing.

3. Drizzle the dressing over the broccoli, apple, and raisin mixture.

4. Gently toss all the ingredients together until well coated with the dressing.

5. Divide the broccoli and apple salad into four serving plates.

6. If desired, sprinkle chopped pecans over the top for added crunch and flavor.

7. Serve immediately as a crisp and satisfying salad.

Nutritional Information (per serving):

- Carbs: 27g

- Fats: 12g

- Fiber: 5g

- Protein: 3g

Beet and Goat Cheese Carpaccio

Prep Time: 15 minutes
Cook Time: 0 minutes
Number of Servings: 4

Ingredients:

- 4 large beets, cooked and peeled

- 4 ounces goat cheese, thinly sliced

- 1/4 cup fresh basil leaves

- 1/4 cup toasted walnuts, chopped
- 2 tablespoons extra-virgin olive oil
- 1 tablespoon balsamic vinegar
- Salt and freshly ground black pepper, to taste
- Fresh basil leaves for garnish (optional)

Instructions:

1. Slice the cooked and peeled beets very thinly using a sharp knife or a mandoline slicer.

2. Arrange the beet slices on four serving plates, slightly overlapping to create a Carpaccio-style presentation.

3. Place the thinly sliced goat cheese evenly over the beet slices.

4. Scatter fresh basil leaves and chopped toasted walnuts over the goat cheese.

5. In a small bowl, whisk the extra-virgin olive oil and balsamic vinegar to make the dressing. Season with salt and freshly ground black pepper to taste.

6. Drizzle the dressing over the beet and goat cheese Carpaccio.

7. If desired, garnish with additional fresh basil leaves.

8. Serve immediately as an elegant and flavorful appetizer or salad.

Nutritional Information (per serving):

- Carbs: 14g
- Fats: 22g
- Fiber: 4g
- Protein: 9g

Cucumber and Red Onion Salad with Yogurt Dressing

Prep Time: 15 minutes
Cook Time: 0 minutes
Number of Servings: 4

Ingredients:

For the Salad:

- 4 cups cucumber, thinly sliced
- 1 small red onion, thinly sliced
- 2 tablespoons fresh dill, chopped
- 1/4 cup crumbled feta cheese (optional)

For the Yogurt Dressing:

- 1 cup Greek yogurt
- 2 tablespoons lemon juice
- 1 tablespoon olive oil
- 1 clove garlic, minced
- Salt and freshly ground black pepper, to taste

Instructions:

1. In a large salad bowl, add the thinly sliced cucumber, thinly sliced red onion, and chopped fresh dill.
2. If desired, sprinkle crumbled feta cheese over the top of the salad.
3. In a separate small bowl, whisk the Greek yogurt, lemon juice, olive oil, minced garlic, salt, and freshly ground black pepper to make the dressing.
4. Drizzle the yogurt dressing over the salad ingredients.
5. Gently toss the salad to ensure it's well coated with the dressing.
6. Divide the cucumber and red onion salad into four serving plates.
7. Serve immediately as a refreshing and creamy salad.

Nutritional Information (per serving):

- Carbs: 10g
- Fats: 10g
- Fiber: 2g
- Protein: 7g

Caprese Salad with Balsamic Reduction

Prep Time: 10 minutes
Cook Time: 10 minutes
Number of Servings: 4

Ingredients:

- 4 large tomatoes, sliced
- 8 ounces fresh mozzarella cheese, sliced
- 1/2 cup fresh basil leaves
- 2 tablespoons extra-virgin olive oil
- Salt and freshly ground black pepper, to taste

For the Balsamic Reduction:

- 1/2 cup balsamic vinegar
- 2 tablespoons honey

Instructions:

1. In a small saucepan, add the balsamic vinegar and honey.

2. Bring the mixture to a boil over medium heat, then reduce the heat to low and simmer for about 10 minutes or until the balsamic vinegar has thickened and reduced by half. Take it out from heat and let it cool.

3. Arrange the sliced tomatoes, fresh mozzarella, and fresh basil leaves on a serving platter, alternating them in a pattern.

4. Drizzle the extra-virgin olive oil over the tomato, mozzarella, and basil.

5. Season the salad with salt and freshly ground black pepper to taste.

6. Drizzle the cooled balsamic reduction over the top of the salad.

7. Serve immediately as a classic and delightful Caprese salad.

Nutritional Information (per serving):

- Carbs: 16g
- Fats: 19g
- Fiber: 2g

- Protein: 15g

Greek Salad with Feta and Olives

Prep Time: 15 minutes
Cook Time: 0 minutes
Number of Servings: 4

Ingredients:

- 4 cups cucumber, diced
- 4 cups tomatoes, diced
- 1 cup red onion, thinly sliced
- 1 cup Kalamata olives, pitted and sliced
- 1 cup feta cheese, crumbled
- 1/4 cup fresh parsley leaves, chopped
- 1/4 cup extra-virgin olive oil
- 2 tablespoons red wine vinegar
- 1 teaspoon dried oregano
- Salt and freshly ground black pepper, to taste

Instructions:

1. In a large salad bowl, add the diced cucumber, diced tomatoes, thinly sliced red onion, sliced Kalamata olives, crumbled feta cheese, and chopped fresh parsley leaves.

2. In a small bowl, whisk the extra-virgin olive oil, red wine vinegar, dried oregano, salt, and freshly ground black pepper to make the dressing.

3. Drizzle the dressing over the Greek salad ingredients.

4. Gently toss the salad to ensure it's well coated with the dressing.

5. Divide the Greek salad into four serving plates.

6. Serve immediately as a flavorful and refreshing salad.

Nutritional Information (per serving):

- Carbs: 16g

- Fats: 32g

- Fiber: 4g

- Protein: 9g

Mandarin Orange Spinach Salad
Prep Time: 15 minutes
Cook Time: 0 minutes
Number of Servings: 4

Ingredients:

- 8 cups fresh spinach leaves, washed and dried

- 1 can (11 ounces) mandarin oranges, drained

- 1/2 cup red onion, thinly sliced

- 1/4 cup sliced almonds, toasted

- 1/4 cup poppy seed dressing

- 2 tablespoons red wine vinegar

- Salt and freshly ground black pepper, to taste

Instructions:

1. In a large salad bowl, place the fresh spinach leaves.

2. Top the spinach with the drained mandarin oranges and thinly sliced red onion.

3. Sprinkle the toasted sliced almonds over the top of the salad.

4. In a small bowl, whisk the poppy seed dressing and red wine vinegar.

5. Drizzle the dressing mixture over the salad.

6. Season the salad with salt and freshly ground black pepper to taste.

7. Gently toss the salad to ensure the ingredients are well coated with the dressing.

8. Divide the Mandarin Orange Spinach Salad into four serving plates.

9. Serve immediately as a sweet and tangy salad.

Nutritional Information (per serving):

- Carbs: 18g

- Fats: 8g

- Fiber: 3g

- Protein: 3g

Roasted Beet and Goat Cheese Salad

Prep Time: 15 minutes
Cook Time: 45 minutes
Number of Servings: 4

Ingredients:

- 4 medium beets, peeled and diced into 1-inch cubes

- 2 tablespoons olive oil

- Salt and freshly ground black pepper, to taste

- 8 cups mixed salad greens (such as arugula and baby spinach)

- 4 ounces goat cheese, crumbled

- 1/4 cup walnuts, toasted and chopped

For the Balsamic Vinaigrette:

- 3 tablespoons balsamic vinegar

- 2 tablespoons extra-virgin olive oil

- 1 teaspoon Dijon mustard

- 1/2 teaspoon honey

- Salt and freshly ground black pepper, to taste

Instructions:

1. Turn on your oven and set it to 400°F (200°C) to preheat.

2. In a large mixing bowl, toss the diced beets with olive oil, salt, and freshly ground black pepper.

3. Spread the seasoned beets in a single layer on a baking sheet.

4. Roast the beets in the preheated oven for about 45 minutes, or until tender and slightly caramelized, stirring once or twice during roasting. Take it out from the oven and let them cool.

5. In a small bowl, whisk the balsamic vinegar, extra-virgin olive oil, Dijon mustard, honey, salt, and freshly ground black pepper to make the vinaigrette.

6. In a large salad bowl, place the mixed salad greens.

7. Top the greens with the roasted beets, crumbled goat cheese, and toasted chopped walnuts.

8. Drizzle the balsamic vinaigrette over the salad.

9. Gently toss the salad to ensure everything is well coated with the dressing.

10. Divide the Roasted Beet and Goat Cheese Salad into four serving plates.

11. Serve immediately as a colorful and flavorful salad.

Nutritional Information (per serving):

- Carbs: 18g

- Fats: 18g

- Fiber: 5g

- Protein: 8g

Quinoa and Chickpea Salad

Prep Time: 15 minutes
Cook Time: 15 minutes
Number of Servings: 4

Ingredients:

- 1 cup quinoa

- 2 cups water

- 1 can (15 ounces) chickpeas, drained and rinsed

- 1 cup cucumber, diced
- 1 cup red bell pepper, diced
- 1/2 cup red onion, finely chopped
- 1/4 cup fresh parsley leaves, chopped
- 1/4 cup fresh lemon juice
- 3 tablespoons extra-virgin olive oil
- 1 teaspoon ground cumin
- 1/2 teaspoon paprika
- Salt and freshly ground black pepper, to taste

Instructions:

1. Rinse the quinoa thoroughly under cold water in a fine-mesh strainer.
2. In a medium saucepan, add the rinsed quinoa and two cups of water. Bring to a boil over high heat.
3. Reduce the heat to low, cover, and simmer for 12-15 minutes, or until the quinoa is tender and the liquid is absorbed.
4. Take out the cooked quinoa from heat and let it cool.
5. In a large mixing bowl, add the cooked and cooled quinoa, drained and rinsed chickpeas, diced cucumber, diced red bell pepper, finely chopped red onion, and chopped fresh parsley leaves.
6. In a separate small bowl, whisk the fresh lemon juice, extra-virgin olive oil, ground cumin, paprika, salt, and freshly ground black pepper to make the dressing.
7. Drizzle the dressing over the quinoa and chickpea salad.
8. Gently toss all the ingredients together until well coated with the dressing.
9. Divide the salad into four serving plates.
10. Serve immediately as a healthy and protein-packed salad.

Nutritional Information (per serving):

- Carbs: 45g

- Fats: 14g

- Fiber: 8g

- Protein: 12g

Waldorf Salad

Prep Time: 20 minutes
Cook Time: 0 minutes
Number of Servings: 4

Ingredients:

- 2 cups apples, diced

- 1 cup celery, thinly sliced

- 1/2 cup red grapes, halved

- 1/2 cup walnut halves, toasted and chopped

- 1/2 cup mayonnaise

- 1/4 cup Greek yogurt

- 1 tablespoon lemon juice

- 1 tablespoon honey

- Salt and freshly ground black pepper, to taste

- Fresh lettuce leaves for serving (optional)

Instructions:

1. In a large mixing bowl, add the diced apples, thinly sliced celery, halved red grapes, and toasted chopped walnut halves.

2. In a separate small bowl, whisk the mayonnaise, Greek yogurt, lemon juice, honey, salt, and freshly ground black pepper to make the dressing.

3. Drizzle the dressing over the Waldorf salad ingredients.

4. Gently toss the salad to ensure everything is well coated with the dressing.

5. If desired, serve the Waldorf Salad on fresh lettuce leaves.

6. Divide the salad into four serving plates.

7. Serve immediately as a classic and refreshing salad.

Nutritional Information (per serving):

- Carbs: 28g
- Fats: 31g
- Fiber: 4g
- Protein: 5g

Tuna Salad with Avocado

Prep Time: 15 minutes
Cook Time: 0 minutes
Number of Servings: 2

Ingredients:

- 2 cans (5 ounces each) tuna in water, drained
- 1 avocado, diced
- 1/4 cup red onion, finely chopped
- 1/4 cup celery, finely chopped
- 2 tablespoons fresh parsley leaves, chopped
- 2 tablespoons mayonnaise
- 1 tablespoon lemon juice
- Salt and freshly ground black pepper, to taste
- Lettuce leaves for serving (optional)

Instructions:

1. In a medium mixing bowl, add the drained tuna, diced avocado, finely chopped red onion, finely chopped celery, and chopped fresh parsley leaves.

2. In a separate small bowl, whisk the mayonnaise, lemon juice, salt, and freshly ground black pepper to make the dressing.

3. Drizzle the dressing over the tuna salad ingredients.

4. Gently toss the salad to ensure everything is well coated with the dressing.

5. If desired, serve the Tuna Salad on lettuce leaves.

6. Divide the salad into two serving plates.

7. Serve immediately as a delicious and creamy salad.

Nutritional Information (per serving):

- Carbs: 12g
- Fats: 25g
- Fiber: 7g
- Protein: 26g

Potato Salad with Dill Dressing

Prep Time: 20 minutes
Cook Time: 15 minutes
Number of Servings: 4

Ingredients:

For the Potato Salad:

- 1.5 pounds potatoes, peeled and diced into bite-sized pieces
- 1/2 cup red onion, finely chopped
- 1/4 cup fresh dill, chopped
- 1/4 cup dill pickles, diced
- 1/4 cup celery, finely chopped
- 2 hard-boiled eggs, chopped (optional)
- Salt and freshly ground black pepper, to taste

For the Dill Dressing:

- 1/2 cup mayonnaise
- 2 tablespoons Greek yogurt
- 2 tablespoons fresh dill, chopped
- 1 tablespoon Dijon mustard

- 1 tablespoon white wine vinegar
- Salt and freshly ground black pepper, to taste

Instructions:

1. Place the diced potatoes in a large pot, cover them with cold water, and add a pinch of salt.

2. Bring the water to a boil over high heat, then reduce the heat to medium and simmer for 10-15 minutes or until the potatoes are tender when pierced with a fork.

3. Drain the potatoes and let them cool to room temperature.

4. In a large mixing bowl, add the cooled diced potatoes, finely chopped red onion, chopped fresh dill, diced dill pickles, chopped celery, and chopped hard-boiled eggs (if using).

5. In a separate small bowl, whisk the mayonnaise, Greek yogurt, chopped fresh dill, Dijon mustard, white wine vinegar, salt, and freshly ground black pepper to make the dressing.

6. Drizzle the dill dressing over the potato salad ingredients.

7. Gently toss the salad to ensure everything is well coated with the dressing.

8. Divide the Potato Salad with Dill Dressing into four serving plates.

9. Serve immediately as a creamy and flavorful salad.

Nutritional Information (per serving):

- Carbs: 37g
- Fats: 27g
- Fiber: 4g
- Protein: 5g

Roasted Sweet Potato Salad

Prep Time: 15 minutes
Cook Time: 30 minutes
Number of Servings: 4

Ingredients:

- 3 large sweet potatoes, peeled and diced into 1-inch cubes
- 2 tablespoons olive oil
- Salt and freshly ground black pepper, to taste
- 1/2 cup red bell pepper, diced
- 1/2 cup red onion, finely chopped
- 1/4 cup fresh parsley leaves, chopped
- 1/4 cup feta cheese, crumbled
- 2 tablespoons balsamic vinegar
- 1 tablespoon honey
- 1 teaspoon Dijon mustard

Instructions:

1. Turn on your oven and set it to 425°F (220°C) to preheat.
2. In a large mixing bowl, toss the diced sweet potatoes with olive oil, salt, and freshly ground black pepper.
3. Spread the seasoned sweet potatoes in a single layer on a baking sheet.
4. Roast the sweet potatoes in the preheated oven for about 30 minutes or until tender and slightly caramelized, stirring once or twice during roasting. Take it out from the oven and let them cool.
5. In a separate small bowl, whisk the balsamic vinegar, honey, and Dijon mustard to make the dressing.
6. In a large salad bowl, place the roasted sweet potatoes, diced red bell pepper, finely chopped red onion, chopped fresh parsley leaves, and crumbled feta cheese.
7. Drizzle the dressing over the salad.
8. Gently toss the salad to ensure everything is well coated with the dressing.
9. Divide the Roasted Sweet Potato Salad into four serving plates.
10. Serve immediately as a delicious and slightly sweet salad.

Nutritional Information (per serving):

- Carbs: 38g

- Fats: 8g

- Fiber: 5g

- Protein: 4g

Cucumber and Tomato Salad with Dijon Dressing

Prep Time: 15 minutes
Cook Time: 0 minutes
Number of Servings: 4

Ingredients:

For the Salad:

- 4 cups cucumber, diced

- 4 cups tomatoes, diced

- 1/2 cup red onion, finely chopped

- 1/4 cup fresh basil leaves, chopped

- Salt and freshly ground black pepper, to taste

For the Dijon Dressing:

- 2 tablespoons Dijon mustard

- 2 tablespoons red wine vinegar

- 1/4 cup extra-virgin olive oil

- 1 clove garlic, minced

- Salt and freshly ground black pepper, to taste

Instructions:

1. In a large salad bowl, add the diced cucumber, diced tomatoes, finely chopped red onion, and chopped fresh basil leaves.

2. In a separate small bowl, whisk the Dijon mustard, red wine vinegar, extra-virgin olive oil, minced garlic, salt, and freshly ground black pepper to make the dressing.

3. Drizzle the Dijon dressing over the salad ingredients.

4. Gently toss the salad to ensure everything is well coated with the dressing.

5. Season the salad with additional salt and freshly ground black pepper to taste if needed.

6. Divide the Cucumber and Tomato Salad into four serving plates.

7. Serve immediately as a fresh and tangy salad.

Nutritional Information (per serving):

- Carbs: 13g

- Fats: 14g

- Fiber: 3g

- Protein: 2g

MAIN DISHES

Lemon Herb Baked Tilapia

Prep Time: 15 minutes
Cook Time: 20 minutes
Servings: 4

Ingredients:

- 4 tilapia fillets (about 6 ounces each)
- 2 tablespoons olive oil
- 2 tablespoons fresh lemon juice
- 2 cloves garlic, minced
- 1 teaspoon dried basil
- 1 teaspoon dried thyme
- 1 teaspoon dried rosemary
- 1/2 teaspoon salt
- 1/4 teaspoon black pepper
- 1 lemon, thinly sliced
- Fresh parsley, for garnish (optional)

Instructions:

1. Turn on your oven and set it to 375°F (190°C) to preheat.
2. In a small bowl, whisk the olive oil, fresh lemon juice, minced garlic, dried basil, dried thyme, dried rosemary, salt, and black pepper.
3. Place the tilapia fillets in a baking dish and pour the lemon herb mixture over them, ensuring each fillet is well coated.
4. Arrange the lemon slices on top of the fillets.
5. Cover the baking dish with aluminum foil and bake in the preheated oven for 15 minutes.

6. After 15 minutes, take out the foil, and continue baking for an extra 5 minutes or until the tilapia flakes easily with a fork and the edges are slightly browned.

7. Garnish with fresh parsley, if desired.

Nutritional Information (Per Serving):

- Carbs: 2 grams

- Fats: 12 grams

- Fiber: 0 grams

- Protein: 31 grams

Balsamic Glazed Chicken Thighs

Prep Time: 10 minutes
Cook Time: 25 minutes
Servings: 4

Ingredients:

- 4 bone-in, skin-on chicken thighs

- 1/4 cup balsamic vinegar

- 2 tablespoons olive oil

- 2 cloves garlic, minced

- 2 tablespoons honey

- 1 teaspoon dried rosemary

- 1/2 teaspoon dried thyme

- Salt and black pepper, to taste

- Fresh parsley, for garnish (optional)

Instructions:

1. Turn on your oven and set it to 375°F (190°C) to preheat.

2. In a small bowl, whisk the balsamic vinegar, olive oil, minced garlic, honey, dried rosemary, dried thyme, salt, and black pepper.

3. Place the chicken thighs in a baking dish and pour the balsamic mixture over them, ensuring well coated.

4. Season the chicken with additional salt and black pepper, if desired.

5. Bake the chicken thighs in the preheated oven for 20-25 minutes or until the chicken is properly cooked, and the skin is crispy, basting the chicken with the balsamic glaze every 10 minutes.

6. If desired, garnish with fresh parsley before serving.

Nutritional Information (Per Serving):

- Carbs: 9 grams

- Fats: 21 grams

- Fiber: 0 grams

- Protein: 24 grams

Pork Medallions with Apple Cider Reduction

Prep Time: 10 minutes
Cook Time: 20 minutes
Servings: 4

Ingredients:

- 1 pound pork tenderloin, cut into 1-inch thick medallions

- 2 tablespoons olive oil

- 1/2 teaspoon salt

- 1/4 teaspoon black pepper

- 2 cloves garlic, minced

- 1 cup apple cider

- 2 tablespoons Dijon mustard

- 1 tablespoon fresh thyme leaves

- 2 tablespoons unsalted butter

Instructions:

1. Season the pork medallions with salt and black pepper.

2. Heat one tablespoon of olive oil in a large skillet over medium-high heat. Add the pork medallions and cook for about 3-4 minutes on

each side or until browned and properly cooked. Take out the pork from the skillet and set it aside.

3. In the same skillet, add the remaining one tablespoon of olive oil and minced garlic. Sauté the garlic for about 30 seconds or until fragrant.

4. Pour in the apple cider and bring it to a boil. Reduce the heat to low and simmer for about 5 minutes or until the cider has reduced by half.

5. Stir in the Dijon mustard and fresh thyme leaves. Cook for an extra 2 minutes, allowing the sauce to thicken.

6. Return the cooked pork medallions to the skillet and simmer for another 2 minutes, turning the pork to coat it evenly with the sauce.

7. Stir in the unsalted butter until it's fully melted and the sauce is glossy.

8. Serve the pork medallions with the apple cider reduction sauce spooned over the top.

Nutritional Information (Per Serving):

- Carbs: 10 grams

- Fats: 15 grams

- Fiber: 0 grams

- Protein: 29 grams

Stuffed Portobello Mushrooms with Quinoa

Prep Time: 15 minutes
Cook Time: 25 minutes
Servings: 4

Ingredients:

- 4 large Portobello mushrooms, stems and gills removed

- 1 cup quinoa

- 2 cups vegetable broth

- 2 tablespoons olive oil

- 1 small onion, finely diced
- 2 cloves garlic, minced
- 1 red bell pepper, diced
- 1 cup baby spinach, chopped
- 1/4 cup grated Parmesan cheese
- 1/4 cup chopped fresh parsley
- Salt and black pepper, to taste

Instructions:

1. Turn on your oven and set it to 375°F (190°C) to preheat.

2. Rinse the quinoa under cold water and drain.

3. In a medium saucepan, add the quinoa and vegetable broth. Bring to a boil, then reduce the heat to low, cover, and simmer for about 15 minutes or until the quinoa is cooked and the liquid is absorbed. Take it out from heat and fluff the quinoa with a fork.

4. While the quinoa is cooking, heat one tablespoon of olive oil in a large skillet over medium heat. Add the diced onion and cook for 2-3 minutes until it becomes translucent.

5. Add the minced garlic and diced red bell pepper to the skillet. Cook for an extra 2-3 minutes until the pepper is tender.

6. Stir in the chopped baby spinach and cook for another 2 minutes or until the spinach is wilted.

7. Combine the cooked quinoa, sautéed vegetable mixture, grated Parmesan cheese, and chopped fresh parsley in a mixing bowl. Season with salt and black pepper to taste. Mix sufficiently.

8. Brush the outside of the Portobello mushrooms with the remaining one tablespoon of olive oil and place them on a baking sheet.

9. Stuff each Portobello mushroom cap with the quinoa mixture, pressing down gently to pack it in.

10. Bake the stuffed Portobello mushrooms in the preheated oven for 20-25 minutes or until the mushrooms are tender and the stuffing is heated through.

11. Serve hot, garnished with additional chopped parsley if desired.

Nutritional Information (Per Serving):

- Carbs: 35 grams

- Fats: 9 grams

- Fiber: 5 grams

- Protein: 10 grams

Turkey and Zucchini Meatballs

Prep Time: 15 minutes
Cook Time: 20 minutes
Servings: 4

Ingredients:

- 1 pound ground turkey

- 2 medium zucchinis, grated and excess moisture squeezed out

- 1/2 cup breadcrumbs

- 1/4 cup grated Parmesan cheese

- 1/4 cup finely chopped fresh parsley

- 1/4 cup finely chopped onion

- 1 egg

- 2 cloves garlic, minced

- 1/2 teaspoon dried oregano

- 1/2 teaspoon dried basil

- Salt and black pepper, to taste

- Olive oil, for cooking

Instructions:

1. In a large mixing bowl, add the ground turkey, grated zucchini, breadcrumbs, grated Parmesan cheese, chopped fresh parsley, finely chopped onion, egg, minced garlic, dried oregano, dried basil, salt, and black pepper. Mix until all ingredients are well combined.

2. Preheat a large skillet over medium-high heat and add a bit of olive oil to prevent sticking.

3. Form the mixture into meatballs, about 1.5 inches in diameter, and place them in the hot skillet. Cook for about 4-5 minutes on each side or until the meatballs are browned and properly cooked.

4. If needed, you can cook the meatballs in batches to avoid overcrowding the skillet.

5. Once the meatballs are cooked, take them out from the skillet and place them on a paper towel-lined plate to drain any excess oil.

6. Serve the turkey and zucchini meatballs hot with your choice of dipping sauce or over pasta or salad.

Nutritional Information (Per Serving):

- Carbs: 13 grams

- Fats: 11 grams

- Fiber: 2 grams

- Protein: 27 grams

Baked Cod with Lemon Dill Sauce

Prep Time: 15 minutes
Cook Time: 20 minutes
Servings: 4

Ingredients:

- 4 cod fillets (about 6 ounces each)

- 2 tablespoons olive oil

- Salt and black pepper, to taste

- 1 lemon, sliced into rounds

- Fresh dill sprigs, for garnish (optional)

Lemon Dill Sauce:

- 1/2 cup mayonnaise

- 1/4 cup sour cream

- 1 lemon, juiced and zested

- 1 tablespoon fresh dill, finely chopped

- 1 clove garlic, minced

- Salt and black pepper, to taste

Instructions:

1. Turn on your oven and set it to 375°F (190°C) to preheat.

2. Pat the cod fillets dry with paper towels and place them on a baking sheet lined with parchment paper or lightly greased.

3. Brush the cod fillets with olive oil and season with salt and black pepper.

4. Arrange lemon slices on top of each cod fillet.

5. Bake the cod in the preheated oven for about 15-20 minutes or until the fish flakes easily with a fork and is opaque throughout.

6. While the cod is baking, prepare the lemon dill sauce. In a small bowl, whisk mayonnaise, sour cream, lemon juice, lemon zest, finely chopped fresh dill, minced garlic, salt, and black pepper. Mix until well combined.

7. Once the cod is done baking, remove it from the oven.

8. Serve the baked cod hot, drizzled with lemon dill sauce, and garnished with fresh dill sprigs if desired.

Nutritional Information (Per Serving):

- Carbs: 4 grams

- Fats: 29 grams

- Fiber: 0 grams

- Protein: 32 grams

Tofu and Vegetable Stir-Fry with Teriyaki Sauce

Prep Time: 15 minutes
Cook Time: 15 minutes
Servings: 4

Ingredients:

- 14 ounces (400 grams) extra-firm tofu, cubed
- 2 tablespoons vegetable oil
- 1 red bell pepper, sliced
- 1 yellow bell pepper, sliced
- 1 cup broccoli florets
- 1 cup snap peas, trimmed
- 1 carrot, julienned
- 3 cloves garlic, minced
- 1 tablespoon fresh ginger, minced
- Sesame seeds, for garnish (optional)

Teriyaki Sauce:

- 1/4 cup low-sodium soy sauce
- 2 tablespoons honey
- 2 tablespoons rice vinegar
- 1 tablespoon mirin
- 1 teaspoon cornstarch

Instructions:

1. Press the tofu: Wrap the tofu in paper towels and place a heavy object (like a cast-iron skillet) on top to remove excess moisture. Let it sit for about 10 minutes. Then, cut the tofu into cubes.

2. In a small bowl, whisk the ingredients for the teriyaki sauce: low-sodium soy sauce, honey, rice vinegar, mirin, and cornstarch. Set aside.

3. Heat one tablespoon of vegetable oil in a large skillet or wok over medium-high heat.

4. Add the tofu cubes to the skillet and cook for 4-5 minutes, turning occasionally, until golden brown on all sides. Take out the tofu from the skillet and set aside.

5. In the same skillet, add the remaining one tablespoon of vegetable oil.

6. Add the minced garlic and minced ginger to the skillet. Stir-fry for about 30 seconds until fragrant.

7. Add the sliced red bell pepper, yellow bell pepper, broccoli florets, snap peas, and julienned carrot to the skillet. Stir-fry for 3-4 minutes until the vegetables are tender-crisp.

8. Return the cooked tofu to the skillet with the stir-fried vegetables.

9. Pour the teriyaki sauce over the tofu and vegetables. Stir-fry for an extra 2 minutes, or until the sauce thickens and coats the tofu and vegetables evenly.

10. Serve the tofu and vegetable stir-fry hot, garnished with sesame seeds if desired.

Nutritional Information (Per Serving):

- Carbs: 25 grams
- Fats: 11 grams
- Fiber: 4 grams
- Protein: 12 grams

Roasted Duck Breast with Orange Glaze

Prep Time: 15 minutes
Cook Time: 30 minutes
Servings: 4

Ingredients:

- 4 duck breast halves
- Salt and black pepper, to taste
- 1 tablespoon olive oil
- 1/2 cup orange juice
- Zest of 1 orange
- 1/4 cup honey
- 2 tablespoons soy sauce
- 2 cloves garlic, minced

- 1 tablespoon fresh rosemary leaves, chopped
- 1 tablespoon fresh thyme leaves, chopped
- Orange slices, for garnish (optional)

Instructions:

1. Turn on your oven and set it to 400°F (200°C) to preheat.

2. Score the skin of the duck breasts in a crisscross pattern, being careful not to cut into the meat. Season both sides of the duck breasts with salt and black pepper.

3. Heat a large ovenproof skillet over medium-high heat. Add the olive oil.

4. Place the duck breasts in the hot skillet, skin-side down. Cook for about 5-6 minutes, or until the skin is browned and crispy. Remove any excess rendered fat from the skillet as needed.

5. Flip the duck breasts and cook for an extra 2 minutes on the other side.

6. Transfer the skillet to the preheated oven and roast the duck breasts for 8-10 minutes for medium-rare or longer if you prefer them more well-done.

7. While the duck is roasting, prepare the orange glaze. In a small saucepan, add the orange juice, orange zest, honey, soy sauce, minced garlic, chopped fresh rosemary, and chopped fresh thyme. Bring the mixture to a simmer and cook for 5-7 minutes, or until the glaze thickens slightly.

8. Take out the duck breasts from the oven and let them rest for a few minutes.

9. Slice the duck breasts and drizzle the orange glaze over the top.

10. Garnish with orange slices if desired and serve hot.

Nutritional Information (Per Serving):

- Carbs: 12 grams
- Fats: 20 grams
- Fiber: 0 grams
- Protein: 30 grams

Beef and Broccoli Stir-Fry

Prep Time: 15 minutes
Cook Time: 15 minutes
Servings: 4

Ingredients:

- 1 pound flank steak, thinly sliced
- 1/2 cup low-sodium soy sauce
- 2 tablespoons brown sugar
- 2 cloves garlic, minced
- 1 tablespoon fresh ginger, minced
- 1 tablespoon cornstarch
- 2 tablespoons vegetable oil
- 4 cups broccoli florets
- 1/2 cup beef broth
- 1 teaspoon sesame oil (optional)
- Cooked rice, for serving
- Sesame seeds, for garnish (optional)

Instructions:

1. In a bowl, whisk the low-sodium soy sauce, brown sugar, minced garlic, minced ginger, and cornstarch to make the sauce. Set it aside.

2. Heat one tablespoon of vegetable oil in a large skillet or wok over high heat.

3. Add the thinly sliced flank steak to the hot skillet. Stir-fry for about 2-3 minutes, or until the beef is browned. Take out the beef from the skillet and set it aside.

4. In the same skillet, add the remaining one tablespoon of vegetable oil.

5. Add the broccoli florets to the skillet and stir-fry for 2-3 minutes, or until they start to become tender.

6. Return the cooked beef to the skillet with the broccoli.

7. Pour in the beef broth and the previously prepared sauce. Stir sufficiently to combine.

8. Cook for an extra 2-3 minutes, or until the sauce thickens and coats the beef and broccoli evenly.

9. If desired, stir in the optional sesame oil for added flavor.

10. Serve the beef and broccoli stir-fry hot over cooked rice.

11. Garnish with sesame seeds if desired.

Nutritional Information (Per Serving):

- Carbs: 15 grams

- Fats: 11 grams

- Fiber: 2 grams

- Protein: 32 grams

Chicken Piccata with Capers

Prep Time: 15 minutes
Cook Time: 20 minutes
Servings: 4

Ingredients:

- 4 boneless, skinless chicken breasts

- Salt and black pepper, to taste

- 1 cup all-purpose flour

- 2 tablespoons olive oil

- 2 tablespoons unsalted butter

- 1/4 cup fresh lemon juice

- 1/2 cup chicken broth

- 1/4 cup capers, drained

- 1/4 cup fresh parsley, chopped

- Lemon slices, for garnish (optional)

Instructions:

1. Season the chicken breasts with salt and black pepper.

2. Place the all-purpose flour in a shallow dish, and dredge each chicken breast in the flour, shaking off any excess.

3. In a large skillet, heat the olive oil over medium-high heat.

4. Add the chicken breasts to the skillet and cook for about 4-5 minutes on each side, or until golden brown and properly cooked. Take out the chicken from the skillet and set it aside.

5. In the same skillet, add the unsalted butter and let it melt.

6. Pour in the fresh lemon juice and chicken broth, stirring to combine. Bring the mixture to a simmer.

7. Add the capers and chopped fresh parsley to the skillet. Cook for an extra 2-3 minutes to allow the sauce to thicken slightly.

8. Return the cooked chicken breasts to the skillet and cook for another 2 minutes, allowing them to heat through and absorb the flavors of the sauce.

9. Serve the chicken piccata hot, garnished with lemon slices if desired.

Nutritional Information (Per Serving):

-   Carbs: 13 grams

-   Fats: 15 grams

-   Fiber: 1 gram

-   Protein: 36 grams

Lemon Herb Grilled Chicken

Prep Time: 10 minutes
Cook Time: 15 minutes
Servings: 4

Ingredients:

-   4 boneless, skinless chicken breasts

-   2 lemons, juiced and zested

- 3 tablespoons olive oil
- 3 cloves garlic, minced
- 2 tablespoons fresh parsley, finely chopped
- 1 tablespoon fresh thyme leaves
- 1 tablespoon fresh rosemary leaves, minced
- Salt and black pepper, to taste

Instructions:

1. In a bowl, add the fresh lemon juice, lemon zest, olive oil, minced garlic, finely chopped fresh parsley, fresh thyme leaves, minced fresh rosemary, salt, and black pepper. Mix sufficiently to create the marinade.

2. Place the chicken breasts in a resealable plastic bag or a shallow dish.

3. Pour the lemon herb marinade over the chicken breasts, ensuring fully coated. Seal the bag or cover the dish and refrigerate for at least 30 minutes, allowing the chicken to marinate. You can marinate it longer for more flavor if desired.

4. Preheat your grill to medium-high heat and oil the grates to prevent sticking.

5. Take out the chicken breasts from the marinade and let any excess drip off.

6. Grill the chicken breasts for about 6-8 minutes on each side, or until fully cooked and have grill marks. The internal temperature should reach 165°F (74°C) to preheat.

7. While grilling, you can baste the chicken with any remaining marinade for extra flavor.

8. Once cooked, take out the chicken from the grill and let it rest for a few minutes before serving.

9. Serve the lemon herb grilled chicken hot, garnished with additional fresh herbs and lemon slices if desired.

Nutritional Information (Per Serving):

- Carbs: 3 grams

- Fats: 12 grams

- Fiber: 1 gram

- Protein: 27 grams

Beef Stroganoff

Prep Time: 15 minutes
Cook Time: 25 minutes
Servings: 4

Ingredients:

- 1 pound beef sirloin or tenderloin, thinly sliced

- Salt and black pepper, to taste

- 2 tablespoons olive oil

- 1 onion, finely chopped

- 2 cloves garlic, minced

- 8 ounces (225 grams) white mushrooms, sliced

- 2 tablespoons all-purpose flour

- 1 cup beef broth

- 2 tablespoons Worcestershire sauce

- 1 tablespoon Dijon mustard

- 1/2 cup sour cream

- 2 tablespoons fresh parsley, chopped

- Cooked egg noodles or rice, for serving

Instructions:

1. Season the thinly sliced beef with salt and black pepper.

2. In a large skillet, heat the olive oil over medium-high heat.

3. Add the sliced beef to the skillet and cook for about 2-3 minutes per side, or until it's browned. Take out the beef from the skillet and set it aside.

4. In the same skillet, add the chopped onion and minced garlic. Sauté for about 2 minutes until the onion becomes translucent.

5. Add the sliced mushrooms to the skillet and cook for an extra 4-5 minutes until they release their moisture and start to brown.

6. Sprinkle the all-purpose flour over the mushroom mixture and stir sufficiently to combine. Cook for 1-2 minutes to take out the raw flour taste.

7. Pour in the beef broth, Worcestershire sauce, and Dijon mustard. Stir constantly until the mixture thickens and comes to a simmer.

8. Return the cooked beef to the skillet and simmer for an extra 5 minutes to heat the beef through.

9. Stir in the sour cream and cook for 1-2 minutes until the sauce is creamy and heated.

10. Season with additional salt and black pepper if needed.

11. Serve the beef stroganoff hot over cooked egg noodles or rice, garnished with chopped fresh parsley.

Nutritional Information (Per Serving):

- Carbs: 8 grams

- Fats: 21 grams

- Fiber: 1 gram

- Protein: 32 grams

Stuffed Bell Peppers with Ground Turkey

Prep Time: 20 minutes
Cook Time: 45 minutes
Servings: 4

Ingredients:

- 4 large bell peppers (any color)

- 1 pound ground turkey

- 1 cup cooked rice

- 1/2 cup onion, finely chopped

- 1/2 cup canned diced tomatoes, drained
- 1/2 cup shredded mozzarella cheese
- 1/2 teaspoon garlic powder
- 1/2 teaspoon dried oregano
- 1/2 teaspoon dried basil
- Salt and black pepper, to taste
- 1 cup tomato sauce

Instructions:

1. Turn on your oven and set it to 350°F (175°C) to preheat.
2. Cut the tops off the bell peppers and take out the seeds and membranes from the inside. Set the bell peppers aside.
3. In a large skillet, cook the ground turkey over medium-high heat until it's no longer pink, breaking it into small pieces as it cooks. Drain any excess fat.
4. In a mixing bowl, add the cooked ground turkey, cooked rice, finely chopped onion, diced tomatoes, shredded mozzarella cheese, garlic powder, dried oregano, dried basil, salt, and black pepper.
5. Stuff each bell pepper with the turkey and rice mixture, pressing down gently to pack it in.
6. Place the stuffed bell peppers in a baking dish.
7. Pour the tomato sauce over the top of the stuffed bell peppers.
8. Cover the baking dish with aluminum foil and bake in the preheated oven for 35-40 minutes or until the peppers are tender.
9. Take out the foil and bake for an extra 5 minutes, allowing the cheese to melt and turn golden brown.
10. Serve the stuffed bell peppers hot.

Nutritional Information (Per Serving):

- Carbs: 23 grams
- Fats: 14 grams
- Fiber: 3 grams

- Protein: 27 grams

Grilled Shrimp with Garlic Butter

Prep Time: 10 minutes
Cook Time: 5 minutes
Servings: 4

Ingredients:

- 1 pound large shrimp, peeled and deveined
- Salt and black pepper, to taste
- 4 cloves garlic, minced
- 4 tablespoons unsalted butter
- 2 tablespoons fresh parsley, chopped
- 1 tablespoon fresh lemon juice
- 1/4 teaspoon red pepper flakes (optional)
- Lemon wedges, for serving (optional)

Instructions:

1. Preheat your grill to medium-high heat.
2. Season the peeled and deveined shrimp with salt and black pepper.
3. In a small saucepan or microwave-safe bowl, melt the unsalted butter.
4. Stir in the minced garlic, chopped fresh parsley, fresh lemon juice, and red pepper flakes (if using) into the melted butter. Mix sufficiently to create the garlic butter sauce.
5. Thread the seasoned shrimp onto skewers, ensuring evenly spaced.
6. Place the shrimp skewers on the preheated grill and cook for about 2-3 minutes per side, or until they turn pink and opaque. Be careful not to overcook the shrimp as they can become tough.
7. During the last minute of grilling, brush the garlic butter sauce generously over the shrimp, allowing it to sizzle and coat the shrimp.

8. Take out the shrimp skewers from the grill and transfer them to a serving platter.

9. Pour any remaining garlic butter sauce over the grilled shrimp.

10. Serve the grilled shrimp hot, garnished with lemon wedges if desired.

Nutritional Information (Per Serving):

- Carbs: 2 grams
- Fats: 11 grams
- Fiber: 0 grams
- Protein: 23 grams

Eggplant Parmesan

Prep Time: 30 minutes
Cook Time: 45 minutes
Servings: 4

Ingredients:

- 2 medium eggplants, peeled and sliced into 1/2-inch rounds
- Salt, for sweating the eggplant
- 2 cups all-purpose flour
- 4 large eggs, beaten
- 2 cups breadcrumbs
- 1/2 cup grated Parmesan cheese
- 2 cups marinara sauce
- 2 cups shredded mozzarella cheese
- 1/4 cup fresh basil leaves, chopped
- 2 tablespoons olive oil
- Black pepper, to taste

Instructions:

1. Place the eggplant slices in a colander and sprinkle them generously with salt. Allow them to sit for about 30 minutes. This helps remove excess moisture and bitterness from the eggplant.

2. Turn on your oven and set it to 375°F (190°C) to preheat.

3. Rinse the salted eggplant slices under cold water and pat them dry with paper towels.

4. Set up a breading station with three shallow dishes: one with flour, one with beaten eggs, and one with a mixture of breadcrumbs, grated Parmesan cheese, and a pinch of black pepper.

5. Dredge each eggplant slice in the flour, shaking off any excess, then dip it in the beaten eggs, and finally coat it in the breadcrumb mixture. Ensure each slice is evenly coated.

6. Heat the olive oil in a large skillet over medium-high heat. In batches, cook the breaded eggplant slices for about 2-3 minutes per side or until golden brown and crispy. Add more oil as needed for frying. Place the cooked slices on a paper towel-lined plate to remove excess oil.

7. In a baking dish, spread a thin layer of marinara sauce. Arrange a layer of fried eggplant slices on top, followed by a layer of shredded mozzarella cheese and chopped fresh basil. Repeat the layers until all the eggplant slices are used, finishing with a layer of cheese and basil on top.

8. Bake the eggplant Parmesan in the preheated oven for about 25-30 minutes, or until the cheese is bubbly and golden brown.

9. Allow the dish to cool slightly before serving. Serve hot.

Nutritional Information (Per Serving):

- Carbs: 46 grams

- Fats: 21 grams

- Fiber: 9 grams

- Protein: 22 grams

Tofu Stir-Fry with Ginger Sauce

Prep Time: 15 minutes
Cook Time: 15 minutes
Servings: 4

Ingredients:

For the Tofu and Vegetables:

- 14 ounces (400 grams) extra-firm tofu, cubed
- 2 tablespoons vegetable oil
- 1 red bell pepper, sliced
- 1 yellow bell pepper, sliced
- 1 cup broccoli florets
- 1 cup snap peas, trimmed
- 1 carrot, julienned
- 3 cloves garlic, minced
- 1 tablespoon fresh ginger, minced

For the Ginger Sauce:

- 1/4 cup low-sodium soy sauce
- 2 tablespoons rice vinegar
- 2 tablespoons honey
- 1 tablespoon cornstarch
- 1/2 teaspoon red pepper flakes (optional)

Instructions:

1. Press the tofu: Wrap the tofu in paper towels and place a heavy object (like a cast-iron skillet) on top to remove excess moisture. Let it sit for about 10 minutes. Then, cut the tofu into cubes.

2. In a small bowl, whisk the ingredients for the ginger sauce: low-sodium soy sauce, rice vinegar, honey, cornstarch, and red pepper flakes (if using). Set aside.

3. Heat one tablespoon of vegetable oil in a large skillet or wok over medium-high heat.

4. Add the tofu cubes to the skillet and cook for 4-5 minutes, turning occasionally, until golden brown on all sides. Take out the tofu from the skillet and set aside.

5. In the same skillet, add the remaining one tablespoon of vegetable oil.

6. Add the minced garlic and minced ginger to the skillet. Stir-fry for about 30 seconds until fragrant.

7. Add the sliced red bell pepper, yellow bell pepper, broccoli florets, snap peas, and julienned carrot to the skillet. Stir-fry for 3-4 minutes until the vegetables are tender-crisp.

8. Return the cooked tofu to the skillet with the stir-fried vegetables.

9. Pour the ginger sauce over the tofu and vegetables. Stir-fry for an extra 2 minutes, or until the sauce thickens and coats the tofu and vegetables evenly.

10. Serve the tofu stir-fry hot, garnished with sesame seeds if desired.

Nutritional Information (Per Serving):

- Carbs: 22 grams

- Fats: 10 grams

- Fiber: 4 grams

- Protein: 10 grams

Pork Tenderloin with Apples
Prep Time: 10 minutes
Cook Time: 30 minutes
Servings: 4

Ingredients:

- 1 pound pork tenderloin

- Salt and black pepper, to taste

- 2 tablespoons olive oil

- 2 apples, peeled, cored, and sliced

- 1 onion, thinly sliced

- 2 cloves garlic, minced
- 1/2 cup chicken broth
- 1/4 cup apple cider or apple juice
- 1/4 cup heavy cream
- 1 teaspoon fresh thyme leaves
- 1 teaspoon fresh rosemary leaves, minced
- 1 tablespoon butter

Instructions:

1. Turn on your oven and set it to 375°F (190°C) to preheat.

2. Season the pork tenderloin with salt and black pepper on all sides.

3. In a large ovenproof skillet, heat the olive oil over medium-high heat.

4. Add the pork tenderloin to the skillet and sear it for 2-3 minutes per side, or until it's browned on all sides. Take out the pork from the skillet and set it aside.

5. In the same skillet, add the sliced apples and thinly sliced onion. Sauté for 3-4 minutes until they begin to soften.

6. Add the minced garlic and keep on cooking for another 30 seconds until fragrant.

7. Pour in the chicken broth and apple cider (or apple juice) to deglaze the skillet, scraping up any browned bits from the bottom.

8. Return the seared pork tenderloin to the skillet, placing it on top of the apples and onions.

9. Transfer the skillet to the preheated oven and roast for about 15-20 minutes, or until the pork reaches an internal temperature of 145°F (63°C) to preheat.

10. Take out the skillet from the oven and transfer the pork to a cutting board to rest.

11. Place the skillet back on the stovetop over medium heat. Stir in the heavy cream, fresh thyme leaves, minced fresh rosemary, and butter. Simmer for a few minutes until the sauce thickens slightly.

12. Slice the rested pork tenderloin into medallions.

13. Serve the sliced pork with the apple and onion mixture and drizzle the creamy sauce over the top.

Nutritional Information (Per Serving):

- Carbs: 15 grams

- Fats: 18 grams

- Fiber: 2 grams

- Protein: 29 grams

Baked Cod with Herbs

Prep Time: 10 minutes
Cook Time: 15 minutes
Servings: 4

Ingredients:

- 4 cod fillets (6-8 ounces each)

- Salt and black pepper, to taste

- 2 tablespoons olive oil

- 2 cloves garlic, minced

- 1 tablespoon fresh parsley, chopped

- 1 tablespoon fresh dill, chopped

- 1 tablespoon fresh chives, chopped

- 1 tablespoon fresh lemon juice

- Lemon wedges, for serving (optional)

Instructions:

1. Turn on your oven and set it to 400°F (200°C) to preheat.

2. Pat the cod fillets dry with paper towels and place them in a baking dish.

3. Season both sides of the cod fillets with salt and black pepper.

4. In a small bowl, add the minced garlic, chopped fresh parsley, chopped fresh dill, and chopped fresh chives.

5. Drizzle the olive oil over the cod fillets.

6. Sprinkle the herb and garlic mixture evenly over the cod fillets.

7. Squeeze fresh lemon juice over the top.

8. Cover the baking dish with aluminum foil.

9. Bake in the preheated oven for about 12-15 minutes, or until the cod is opaque and flakes easily with a fork.

10. Take out the foil and broil for an extra 2-3 minutes until the top is lightly browned.

11. Serve the baked cod hot, garnished with lemon wedges if desired.

Nutritional Information (Per Serving):

- Carbs: 1 gram

- Fats: 8 grams

- Fiber: 0 grams

- Protein: 33 grams

Zucchini Noodles with Pesto

Prep Time: 15 minutes
Cook Time: 5 minutes
Servings: 4

Ingredients:

- 4 medium zucchinis, spiralized into noodles

- Salt and black pepper, to taste

- 2 tablespoons olive oil

- 1/2 cup prepared pesto sauce

- 1/4 cup grated Parmesan cheese

- 1/4 cup pine nuts, toasted

- Fresh basil leaves, for garnish (optional)

Instructions:

1. Spiralize the zucchinis into noodles using a spiralizer. If you don't have a spiralizer, you can use a vegetable peeler to create long, thin strips. Season the zucchini noodles with salt and black pepper to taste.

2. Heat the olive oil in a large skillet over medium-high heat.

3. Add the zucchini noodles to the skillet and sauté for 2-3 minutes, tossing gently with tongs, until just tender. Be careful not to overcook them; they should still have a slight crunch.

4. Take out the skillet from heat.

5. Stir in the prepared pesto sauce and toss until the zucchini noodles are evenly coated.

6. Sprinkle the grated Parmesan cheese over the top and toss again to combine.

7. Toast the pine nuts in a dry pan over medium heat for about 2-3 minutes, stirring frequently until lightly golden.

8. Serve the zucchini noodles with pesto hot, garnished with toasted pine nuts and fresh basil leaves if desired.

Nutritional Information (Per Serving):

- Carbs: 10 grams
- Fats: 28 grams
- Fiber: 2 grams
- Protein: 7 grams

SIDES

Creamed Cauliflower Recipe

Prep Time: 15 minutes

Cook Time: 20 minutes

Servings: 4

Ingredients:

- 1 large head of cauliflower, cut into florets
- 2 tablespoons unsalted butter
- 2 cloves garlic, minced
- 1/2 cup heavy cream
- 1/4 cup grated Parmesan cheese
- Salt and pepper to taste
- Fresh chives, for garnish

Instructions:

1. Place the cauliflower florets in a large pot and cover them with water. Add a pinch of salt to the water. Bring the water to a boil over high heat, then reduce the heat to medium and simmer the cauliflower for about 10-12 minutes, or until it becomes tender.

2. While the cauliflower is cooking, melt the butter in a separate saucepan over medium heat. Add the minced garlic and sauté for 1-2 minutes, or until fragrant.

3. Drain the cooked cauliflower thoroughly and transfer it to a food processor.

4. Pour the melted garlic butter, heavy cream, and grated Parmesan cheese into the food processor with the cauliflower.

5. Blend the mixture until smooth and creamy, scraping down the sides of the processor as needed to ensure even mixing. You may need to add a splash of water or more cream if the mixture is too thick.

6. Return the creamy cauliflower mixture to the saucepan and heat it over low heat, stirring constantly, for about 3-5 minutes, or until it's heated through.

7. Season the creamed cauliflower with salt and pepper to taste. Adjust the seasoning according to your preferences.

8. Serve the creamed cauliflower hot, garnished with fresh chives.

Nutritional Information (per serving):

- Carbs: 11g

- Fats: 19g

- Fiber: 3g

- Protein: 6g

Lemon Garlic Roasted Broccolini Recipe

Prep Time: 10 minutes

Cook Time: 15 minutes

Servings: 4

Ingredients:

- 1 bunch broccolini, trimmed

- 2 tablespoons olive oil

- 2 cloves garlic, minced

- Zest of 1 lemon

- 2 tablespoons fresh lemon juice

- Salt and pepper to taste

- Grated Parmesan cheese (optional, for garnish)

Instructions:

1. Turn on your oven and set it to 425°F (220°C) to preheat and line a baking sheet with parchment paper.

2. In a small bowl, add the olive oil, minced garlic, lemon zest, and fresh lemon juice. Mix sufficiently.

3. Place the trimmed broccolini on the prepared baking sheet.

4. Drizzle the lemon-garlic mixture over the broccolini, ensuring it's evenly coated.

5. Season the broccolini with salt and pepper to taste.

6. Roast the broccolini in the preheated oven for about 12-15 minutes, or until it becomes tender and slightly crispy at the edges. You can toss it once halfway through the roasting time for even cooking.

7. Take out the roasted broccolini from the oven and transfer it to a serving platter.

8. If desired, garnish the broccolini with grated Parmesan cheese.

9. Serve the Lemon Garlic Roasted Broccolini hot as a delicious side dish.

Nutritional Information (per serving):

- Carbs: 6g

- Fats: 7g

- Fiber: 2g

- Protein: 2g

Miso Glazed Eggplant Recipe

Prep Time: 15 minutes

Cook Time: 25 minutes

Servings: 4

Ingredients:

- 2 large eggplants, sliced into 1/2-inch thick rounds

- 2 tablespoons white miso paste

- 2 tablespoons mirin

- 2 tablespoons soy sauce

- 2 tablespoons rice vinegar

- 2 tablespoons honey

- 1 tablespoon sesame oil

- 2 cloves garlic, minced

- 1 tablespoon grated fresh ginger

- Sesame seeds, for garnish

- Sliced green onions, for garnish

- Cooked white rice, for serving

Instructions:

1. Turn on your oven and set it to 400°F (200°C) to preheat and line a baking sheet with parchment paper.

2. In a small bowl, whisk the white miso paste, mirin, soy sauce, rice vinegar, honey, sesame oil, minced garlic, and grated fresh ginger until you have a smooth glaze.

3. Place the eggplant rounds on the prepared baking sheet.

4. Brush both sides of the eggplant rounds generously with the miso glaze.

5. Roast the eggplant in the preheated oven for about 20-25 minutes, or until it becomes tender and slightly caramelized. You can flip the eggplant rounds halfway through the roasting time for even glazing.

6. While the eggplant is roasting, prepare your cooked white rice according to package instructions.

7. Once the eggplant is done, remove it from the oven.

8. Serve the Miso Glazed Eggplant hot over cooked white rice.

9. Garnish with sesame seeds and sliced green onions.

Nutritional Information (per serving):

- Carbs: 29g

- Fats: 6g

- Fiber: 4g

- Protein: 3g

Ginger Soy Glazed Carrots Recipe

Prep Time: 10 minutes

Cook Time: 20 minutes

Servings: 4

Ingredients:

- 1 pound carrots, peeled and sliced into 1/4-inch thick rounds
- 2 tablespoons soy sauce
- 2 tablespoons honey
- 1 tablespoon grated fresh ginger
- 1 tablespoon unsalted butter
- 1 tablespoon vegetable oil
- Sesame seeds, for garnish
- Chopped fresh cilantro, for garnish

Instructions:

1. In a small bowl, whisk the soy sauce, honey, and grated fresh ginger to make the glaze.
2. Heat a large skillet over medium-high heat and add the vegetable oil and butter.
3. Once the butter has melted and the skillet is hot, add the sliced carrots.
4. Sauté the carrots for about 5 minutes, stirring occasionally, until they start to become tender.
5. Pour the prepared ginger soy glaze over the carrots.
6. Keep on cooking the carrots, stirring frequently, for another 10-15 minutes, or until tender and the glaze has thickened and coated the carrots.
7. Take out the skillet from heat.
8. Transfer the Ginger Soy Glazed Carrots to a serving dish.
9. Garnish with sesame seeds and chopped fresh cilantro.

10. Serve the glazed carrots as a delicious side dish.

Nutritional Information (per serving):

- Carbs: 19g

- Fats: 4g

- Fiber: 3g

- Protein: 1g

Creamy Polenta Cakes Recipe

Prep Time: 15 minutes

Cook Time: 25 minutes

Servings: 4

Ingredients:

- 1 cup yellow cornmeal

- 4 cups water

- 1 teaspoon salt

- 1/2 cup grated Parmesan cheese

- 2 tablespoons unsalted butter

- 1/4 cup heavy cream

- 1/4 cup finely chopped fresh parsley

- 2 cloves garlic, minced

- Olive oil, for frying

- Salt and pepper to taste

Instructions:

1. In a medium saucepan, bring 4 cups of water to a boil.

2. Slowly pour the cornmeal into the boiling water, whisking constantly to avoid lumps.

3. Reduce the heat to low and keep on cooking, stirring frequently, for about 20 minutes, or until the polenta is thick and creamy.

4. Stir in the salt, grated Parmesan cheese, unsalted butter, heavy cream, finely chopped fresh parsley, and minced garlic. Mix sufficiently until all the ingredients are fully incorporated.

5. Transfer the creamy polenta mixture to a greased 9x9-inch baking dish or a similar-sized container. Smooth the top with a spatula.

6. Let the polenta cool and set for at least 30 minutes, or until it's firm.

7. Once the polenta has set, use a round cookie cutter or a glass to cut out individual polenta cakes.

8. Heat a skillet over medium-high heat and add enough olive oil to coat the bottom.

9. Carefully place the polenta cakes in the hot skillet and fry them for about 2-3 minutes on each side, or until they become crispy and golden brown.

10. Take out the polenta cakes from the skillet and place them on a paper towel-lined plate to remove excess oil.

11. Season the Creamy Polenta Cakes with salt and pepper to taste.

12. Serve the polenta cakes hot as a delightful side dish or appetizer.

Nutritional Information (per serving):

- Carbs: 30g
- Fats: 16g
- Fiber: 2g
- Protein: 6g

Roasted Buttery Turnips Recipe

Prep Time: 10 minutes

Cook Time: 30 minutes

Servings: 4

Ingredients:

- 6 medium-sized turnips, peeled and cut into 1-inch cubes
- 2 tablespoons unsalted butter, melted

- 1 tablespoon olive oil
- 2 cloves garlic, minced
- 1 teaspoon dried thyme
- Salt and pepper to taste
- Chopped fresh parsley, for garnish

Instructions:

1. Turn on your oven and set it to 425°F (220°C) to preheat and line a baking sheet with parchment paper.

2. In a large bowl, add the cubed turnips, melted unsalted butter, olive oil, minced garlic, dried thyme, salt, and pepper. Toss everything together until the turnips are evenly coated with the mixture.

3. Spread the seasoned turnips in a single layer on the prepared baking sheet.

4. Roast the turnips in the preheated oven for about 25-30 minutes, or until tender and golden brown. You can stir or flip them halfway through the roasting time for even cooking.

5. Once the turnips are done, take them out from the oven.

6. Transfer the Roasted Buttery Turnips to a serving dish and garnish with chopped fresh parsley.

7. Serve the delicious roasted turnips as a flavorful side dish.

Nutritional Information (per serving):

- Carbs: 10g
- Fats: 8g
- Fiber: 2g
- Protein: 1g

Parmesan Zucchini Rounds Recipe

Prep Time: 10 minutes

Cook Time: 20 minutes

Servings: 4

Ingredients:

- 4 medium zucchini, sliced into 1/4-inch thick rounds
- 1/2 cup grated Parmesan cheese
- 1/4 cup breadcrumbs
- 1/2 teaspoon garlic powder
- 1/2 teaspoon onion powder
- 1/4 teaspoon dried oregano
- 1/4 teaspoon dried basil
- Salt and pepper to taste
- Olive oil cooking spray

Instructions:

1. Turn on your oven and set it to 425°F (220°C) to preheat and line a baking sheet with parchment paper.

2. In a bowl, add the grated Parmesan cheese, breadcrumbs, garlic powder, onion powder, dried oregano, dried basil, salt, and pepper. Mix sufficiently to create the coating mixture.

3. Place the zucchini rounds in a separate bowl.

4. Lightly coat the zucchini rounds with olive oil cooking spray, ensuring evenly coated.

5. Take each zucchini round and press it into the Parmesan breadcrumb mixture, coating both sides generously. Place the coated zucchini rounds on the prepared baking sheet in a single layer.

6. Once all the zucchini rounds are coated and arranged on the baking sheet, lightly spray the tops with olive oil cooking spray.

7. Bake in the preheated oven for about 18-20 minutes, or until the zucchini rounds are tender and the coating is golden brown and crispy.

8. Take out the Parmesan Zucchini Rounds from the oven and let them cool for a minute or two before serving.

9. Serve as a tasty side dish or appetizer.

Nutritional Information (per serving):

- Carbs: 8g

- Fats: 6g

- Fiber: 2g

- Protein: 6g

Cabbage and Bacon Saute Recipe

Prep Time: 10 minutes

Cook Time: 20 minutes

Servings: 4

Ingredients:

- 6 slices bacon, chopped

- 1 small head cabbage, thinly sliced

- 1 onion, thinly sliced

- 2 cloves garlic, minced

- 1/4 teaspoon red pepper flakes (optional)

- Salt and pepper to taste

- Chopped fresh parsley, for garnish

Instructions:

1. In a large skillet, cook the chopped bacon over medium-high heat until it becomes crispy, about 5-7 minutes. Take out the crispy bacon from the skillet and place it on a paper towel-lined plate to drain excess grease. Set aside.

2. In the same skillet, add the thinly sliced cabbage and onion. Cook them over medium heat for about 10-12 minutes, or until they become tender and start to caramelize. Stir occasionally to prevent sticking.

3. Add the minced garlic and red pepper flakes (if using) to the skillet. Sauté for an extra 1-2 minutes, or until the garlic becomes fragrant.

4. Return the crispy bacon to the skillet with the cabbage and onions. Mix everything together.

5. Season the Cabbage and Bacon Saute with salt and pepper to taste. Adjust the seasoning to your preference.

6. Keep on cooking for another 2-3 minutes to ensure everything is heated through and well combined.

7. Take out the skillet from heat.

8. Garnish the sautéed cabbage and bacon with chopped fresh parsley.

9. Serve hot as a delicious side dish or enjoy it as a main course.

Nutritional Information (per serving):

- Carbs: 7g
- Fats: 11g
- Fiber: 2g
- Protein: 5g

Sautéed Swiss Chard with Lemon Recipe

Prep Time: 10 minutes

Cook Time: 10 minutes

Servings: 4

Ingredients:

- 1 bunch Swiss chard, stems removed and leaves sliced into thin strips
- 2 tablespoons olive oil
- 2 cloves garlic, minced
- Zest of 1 lemon
- Juice of 1 lemon
- Salt and pepper to taste

Instructions:

1. Start by washing the Swiss chard thoroughly. Take out the stems and discard them, then slice the leaves into thin strips.

2. Heat the olive oil in a large skillet over medium heat.

3. Add the minced garlic to the skillet and sauté for about 1 minute, or until it becomes fragrant.

4. Add the sliced Swiss chard to the skillet. Sauté for 3-4 minutes, or until the chard begins to wilt and turn bright green.

5. Zest the lemon directly over the skillet and squeeze the juice of the lemon into the pan as well.

6. Continue to sauté for an extra 2-3 minutes, or until the Swiss chard is tender and has absorbed the lemon flavor.

7. Season the Sautéed Swiss Chard with Lemon with salt and pepper to taste. Adjust the seasoning according to your preference.

8. Take out the skillet from heat.

9. Transfer the sautéed Swiss chard to a serving dish.

10. Serve hot as a delightful and vibrant side dish.

Nutritional Information (per serving):

- Carbs: 5g

- Fats: 7g

- Fiber: 1g

- Protein: 1g

Celeriac and Potato Mash Recipe

Prep Time: 15 minutes

Cook Time: 25 minutes

Servings: 4

Ingredients:

- 1 large celeriac (celery root), peeled and diced into 1-inch pieces

- 2 large russet potatoes, peeled and diced into 1-inch pieces

- 4 cups water
- 2 tablespoons unsalted butter
- 1/4 cup heavy cream
- Salt and pepper to taste
- Chopped fresh chives, for garnish

Instructions:

1. In a large pot, add the diced celeriac and potatoes.

2. Add 4 cups of water to the pot, ensuring that the vegetables are submerged. Add a pinch of salt.

3. Bring the water to a boil over high heat, then reduce the heat to medium and simmer for about 15-20 minutes, or until the celeriac and potatoes are fork-tender.

4. Drain the cooked celeriac and potatoes thoroughly.

5. Return the drained celeriac and potatoes to the pot.

6. Add the unsalted butter and heavy cream to the pot.

7. Mash the celeriac and potatoes using a potato masher or a hand mixer until you achieve your desired level of smoothness. Add more cream if needed for a creamier consistency.

8. Season the Celeriac and Potato Mash with salt and pepper to taste. Adjust the seasoning to your preference.

9. Transfer the mashed celeriac and potatoes to a serving dish.

10. Garnish with chopped fresh chives.

11. Serve hot as a comforting and creamy side dish.

Nutritional Information (per serving):

- Carbs: 30g
- Fats: 9g
- Fiber: 4g
- Protein: 3g

Mashed Potatoes Recipe

Prep Time: 15 minutes

Cook Time: 20 minutes

Servings: 4

Ingredients:

- 4 large russet potatoes, peeled and cut into 1-inch cubes
- 4 cups water
- 1/2 cup whole milk
- 4 tablespoons unsalted butter
- Salt and pepper to taste
- Chopped fresh chives, for garnish (optional)

Instructions:

1. Place the peeled and cubed russet potatoes in a large pot.
2. Add 4 cups of water to the pot, ensuring that the potatoes are submerged. Add a pinch of salt.
3. Bring the water to a boil over high heat, then reduce the heat to medium and simmer for about 15-20 minutes, or until the potatoes are fork-tender.
4. Drain the cooked potatoes thoroughly.
5. Return the drained potatoes to the pot.
6. Add the whole milk and unsalted butter to the pot.
7. Mash the potatoes using a potato masher or a hand mixer until smooth and creamy. Add more milk if needed for your desired consistency.
8. Season the Mashed Potatoes with salt and pepper to taste. Adjust the seasoning to your preference.
9. Transfer the mashed potatoes to a serving bowl.
10. Garnish with chopped fresh chives if desired.
11. Serve hot as a classic and comforting side dish.

Nutritional Information (per serving):

- Carbs: 35g

- Fats: 13g

- Fiber: 3g

- Protein: 5g

Garlic Roasted Asparagus Recipe

Prep Time: 10 minutes

Cook Time: 15 minutes

Servings: 4

Ingredients:

- 1 pound fresh asparagus spears, woody ends trimmed

- 2 tablespoons olive oil

- 4 cloves garlic, minced

- Salt and pepper to taste

- Grated Parmesan cheese, for garnish (optional)

- Lemon wedges, for serving (optional)

Instructions:

1. Turn on your oven and set it to 425°F (220°C) to preheat and line a baking sheet with parchment paper.

2. Place the trimmed asparagus spears on the prepared baking sheet.

3. Drizzle the olive oil over the asparagus.

4. Sprinkle the minced garlic evenly over the asparagus.

5. Season the asparagus with salt and pepper to taste.

6. Toss the asparagus spears to ensure well coated with the olive oil, garlic, salt, and pepper.

7. Spread the seasoned asparagus out in a single layer on the baking sheet.

8. Roast in the preheated oven for about 12-15 minutes, or until the asparagus becomes tender and slightly crispy at the tips. You can shake the pan or flip the asparagus halfway through the roasting time for even cooking.

9. Take out the Garlic Roasted Asparagus from the oven.

10. If desired, garnish with grated Parmesan cheese.

11. Serve hot with optional lemon wedges for extra flavor.

Nutritional Information (per serving):

- Carbs: 4g
- Fats: 7g
- Fiber: 2g
- Protein: 2g

Creamed Spinach Recipe

Prep Time: 10 minutes

Cook Time: 15 minutes

Servings: 4

Ingredients:

- 1 pound fresh spinach, washed and trimmed
- 2 tablespoons unsalted butter
- 2 cloves garlic, minced
- 2 tablespoons all-purpose flour
- 1 cup whole milk
- 1/4 teaspoon ground nutmeg
- Salt and pepper to taste
- 1/4 cup grated Parmesan cheese
- 1/4 cup heavy cream

Instructions:

1. Begin by washing and trimming the fresh spinach. Remove any tough stems and roughly chop the leaves.

2. In a large pot or skillet, melt the unsalted butter over medium heat.

3. Add the minced garlic to the melted butter and sauté for about 1 minute, or until it becomes fragrant.

4. Sprinkle the all-purpose flour evenly over the garlic and butter. Stir constantly and cook for another 1-2 minutes to make a roux.

5. Gradually pour in the whole milk while continuously stirring to avoid lumps. Keep stirring until the mixture thickens, which should take about 3-5 minutes.

6. Add the ground nutmeg, salt, and pepper to the creamy mixture. Stir sufficiently to combine.

7. Add the chopped spinach to the pot. Stir gently to coat the spinach with the creamy sauce.

8. Cover the pot and let the spinach wilt for about 3-5 minutes, stirring occasionally. The spinach should become tender and reduce in volume.

9. Stir in the grated Parmesan cheese and heavy cream. Keep on cooking for another 2-3 minutes, or until the Creamed Spinach is heated through and creamy.

10. Adjust the seasoning with additional salt and pepper if needed.

11. Serve hot as a delicious and creamy side dish.

Nutritional Information (per serving):

- Carbs: 9g
- Fats: 14g
- Fiber: 2g
- Protein: 6g

Buttery Corn on the Cob Recipe

Prep Time: 10 minutes

Cook Time: 10 minutes

Servings: 4

Ingredients:

- 4 ears of fresh corn on the cob, husks and silk removed
- 4 tablespoons unsalted butter
- Salt and pepper to taste
- Chopped fresh parsley, for garnish (optional)

Instructions:

1. Start by bringing a large pot of water to a boil. Add a pinch of salt to the boiling water.

2. Carefully add the fresh corn on the cob to the boiling water. Boil for about 5-7 minutes, or until the corn kernels are tender.

3. While the corn is boiling, melt the unsalted butter in a small saucepan over low heat. Keep it warm but not boiling.

4. Once the corn is tender, take out the ears from the boiling water and let them drain briefly.

5. Place each ear of corn on a serving plate.

6. Drizzle the melted unsalted butter over the hot corn.

7. Season the Buttery Corn on the Cob with salt and pepper to taste. Adjust the seasoning according to your preference.

8. If desired, garnish with chopped fresh parsley for added flavor and color.

9. Serve hot as a classic and delicious side dish.

Nutritional Information (per serving):

- Carbs: 24g
- Fats: 12g
- Fiber: 3g
- Protein: 3g

Roasted Brussels Sprouts Recipe

Prep Time: 10 minutes

Cook Time: 25 minutes

Servings: 4

Ingredients:

- 1 pound fresh Brussels sprouts, trimmed and halved
- 2 tablespoons olive oil
- Salt and pepper to taste
- 2 cloves garlic, minced
- 1/4 cup grated Parmesan cheese (optional)

Instructions:

1. Turn on your oven and set it to 425°F (220°C) to preheat and line a baking sheet with parchment paper.

2. In a large bowl, toss the trimmed and halved Brussels sprouts with olive oil, ensuring well coated.

3. Season the Brussels sprouts with salt and pepper to taste. Toss again to distribute the seasoning evenly.

4. Spread the seasoned Brussels sprouts out on the prepared baking sheet in a single layer.

5. Roast in the preheated oven for about 20-25 minutes, or until the Brussels sprouts are tender and have developed a nice caramelized exterior. You can shake the pan or flip the sprouts halfway through the roasting time for even cooking.

6. During the last 5 minutes of roasting, add the minced garlic to the Brussels sprouts and toss to combine. This will infuse them with a delicious garlic flavor.

7. If desired, sprinkle grated Parmesan cheese over the roasted Brussels sprouts as soon as they come out of the oven. The heat will melt the cheese.

8. Serve hot as a delightful and savory side dish.

Nutritional Information (per serving, without Parmesan cheese):

- Carbs: 10g

- Fats: 7g

- Fiber: 4g

- Protein: 3g

Glazed Carrots Recipe

Prep Time: 10 minutes

Cook Time: 15 minutes

Servings: 4

Ingredients:

- 1 pound carrots, peeled and sliced into 1/4-inch thick rounds

- 2 tablespoons unsalted butter

- 1/4 cup brown sugar

- 1/4 cup water

- 1/4 teaspoon salt

- 1/4 teaspoon ground cinnamon

- 1/4 teaspoon ground nutmeg

Instructions:

1. Begin by peeling the carrots and slicing them into 1/4-inch thick rounds.

2. In a large skillet or saucepan, melt the unsalted butter over medium heat.

3. Add the sliced carrots to the melted butter and sauté for about 5 minutes, or until they begin to soften slightly.

4. In a separate bowl, add the brown sugar, water, salt, ground cinnamon, and ground nutmeg. Mix sufficiently to create the glaze.

5. Pour the glaze mixture over the sautéed carrots in the skillet.

6. Stir the carrots and glaze together to ensure well coated.

7. Bring the mixture to a gentle simmer.

8. Reduce the heat to low, cover the skillet, and let the carrots simmer for about 8-10 minutes, or until tender and the glaze has thickened.

9. Check the carrots for doneness by piercing them with a fork; they should be tender but not mushy.

10. Once the carrots are cooked to your liking, take out the Glazed Carrots from the heat.

11. Serve hot as a sweet and savory side dish.

Nutritional Information (per serving):

- Carbs: 23g

- Fats: 6g

- Fiber: 3g

- Protein: 1g

Sautéed Green Beans with Almonds Recipe

Prep Time: 10 minutes

Cook Time: 10 minutes

Servings: 4

Ingredients:

- 1 pound fresh green beans, trimmed

- 2 tablespoons unsalted butter

- 1/4 cup slivered almonds

- 2 cloves garlic, minced

- Salt and pepper to taste

- Lemon wedges, for serving (optional)

Instructions:

1. Begin by trimming the ends of the fresh green beans.

2. In a large skillet, melt the unsalted butter over medium heat.

3. Add the slivered almonds to the melted butter and sauté for about 2-3 minutes, or until the almonds turn golden brown. Stir frequently to prevent burning.

4. Once the almonds are toasted, take them out from the skillet and set them aside.

5. In the same skillet, add the trimmed green beans.

6. Sauté the green beans in the butter and almond remnants for about 5-7 minutes, or until they become tender but still slightly crisp. Stir occasionally.

7. Add the minced garlic to the skillet with the green beans. Sauté for an extra 1-2 minutes, or until the garlic becomes fragrant.

8. Season the Sautéed Green Beans with Almonds with salt and pepper to taste. Adjust the seasoning according to your preference.

9. Return the toasted almonds to the skillet with the green beans. Toss everything together to combine.

10. If desired, serve the green beans with lemon wedges for added flavor.

11. Serve hot as a delightful and crunchy side dish.

Nutritional Information (per serving):

- Carbs: 8g

- Fats: 9g

- Fiber: 4g

- Protein: 3g

Sweet Potato Casserole Recipe

Prep Time: 20 minutes

Cook Time: 45 minutes

Servings: 8

Ingredients:

- 4 cups mashed sweet potatoes (about 4-5 medium sweet potatoes, cooked and peeled)

- 1/2 cup granulated sugar

- 2 large eggs, beaten

- 1/2 cup whole milk

- 1/2 cup unsalted butter, melted

- 1 teaspoon vanilla extract

- 1/2 teaspoon salt

- 1/2 cup packed brown sugar

- 1/2 cup all-purpose flour

- 1/4 cup unsalted butter, melted

- 1 cup chopped pecans

Instructions:

1. Begin by preheating your oven to 350°F (175°C) to preheat and greasing a 9x13-inch baking dish.

2. In a large mixing bowl, add the mashed sweet potatoes, granulated sugar, beaten eggs, whole milk, melted unsalted butter, vanilla extract, and salt. Mix sufficiently until all the ingredients are fully combined.

3. Transfer the sweet potato mixture into the greased baking dish and spread it out evenly.

4. In a separate bowl, prepare the topping by combining the packed brown sugar, all-purpose flour, melted unsalted butter, and chopped pecans. Mix until the topping is crumbly.

5. Sprinkle the pecan topping evenly over the sweet potato mixture in the baking dish.

6. Bake in the preheated oven for about 45 minutes, or until the top is golden brown and the casserole is set in the middle.

7. Take out the Sweet Potato Casserole from the oven and let it cool for a few minutes before serving.

8. Serve hot as a delicious and comforting side dish, especially for holiday meals.

Nutritional Information (per serving):

- Carbs: 50g
- Fats: 30g
- Fiber: 3g
- Protein: 4g

Cucumber Slices with Dill Recipe

Prep Time: 10 minutes

Cook Time: 0 minutes

Servings: 4

Ingredients:

- 2 large cucumbers, thinly sliced
- 1/2 cup sour cream
- 2 tablespoons fresh dill, chopped
- 1 tablespoon white wine vinegar
- Salt and pepper to taste

Instructions:

1. Begin by washing the cucumbers thoroughly. If desired, you can peel them, but it's not necessary.

2. Slice the cucumbers into thin rounds.

3. In a mixing bowl, add the sour cream, chopped fresh dill, and white wine vinegar. Mix until all the ingredients are well incorporated.

4. Season the sour cream mixture with salt and pepper to taste. Adjust the seasoning according to your preference.

5. Add the thinly sliced cucumbers to the sour cream mixture.

6. Gently toss the cucumbers with the dill-infused sour cream until well coated.

7. Refrigerate the Cucumber Slices with Dill for about 15-30 minutes before serving. Chilling allows the flavors to meld together.

8. Serve cold as a refreshing and creamy side dish or salad.

Nutritional Information (per serving):

- Carbs: 6g
- Fats: 7g
- Fiber: 1g
- Protein: 1g

Roasted Cauliflower with Parmesan Recipe

Prep Time: 10 minutes

Cook Time: 25 minutes

Servings: 4

Ingredients:

- 1 large head of cauliflower, cut into florets
- 2 tablespoons olive oil
- 1/2 cup grated Parmesan cheese
- 1 teaspoon garlic powder
- 1 teaspoon onion powder
- Salt and pepper to taste
- Chopped fresh parsley, for garnish (optional)

Instructions:

1. Start by preheating your oven to 425°F (220°C) to preheat and lining a baking sheet with parchment paper.
2. Cut the large head of cauliflower into bite-sized florets. You can remove any tough stems.
3. In a large mixing bowl, toss the cauliflower florets with olive oil until evenly coated.
4. Season the cauliflower with garlic powder, onion powder, salt, and pepper. Toss again to distribute the seasoning evenly.
5. Spread the seasoned cauliflower out on the prepared baking sheet in a single layer.

6. Roast the cauliflower in the preheated oven for about 20-25 minutes, or until the florets are tender and have developed a nice golden brown color. You can shake the pan or flip the cauliflower halfway through the roasting time for even cooking.

7. During the last few minutes of roasting, sprinkle the grated Parmesan cheese evenly over the cauliflower. Return the cauliflower to the oven and roast for an extra 2-3 minutes, or until the cheese is melted and slightly crispy.

8. Take out the Roasted Cauliflower with Parmesan from the oven.

9. If desired, garnish with chopped fresh parsley for added flavor and presentation.

10. Serve hot as a delightful and cheesy side dish.

Nutritional Information (per serving):

- Carbs: 8g
- Fats: 9g
- Fiber: 3g
- Protein: 7g

SNACKS

Baked Cheese Crisps
Prep Time: 10 minutes
Cook Time: 15 minutes
Number of Servings: 4

Ingredients:

- 2 cups shredded Cheddar cheese
- 2 cups shredded Parmesan cheese
- 1 teaspoon garlic powder
- 1 teaspoon onion powder
- 1/2 teaspoon paprika
- 1/4 teaspoon black pepper

Instructions:

1. Turn on your oven and set it to 375°F (190°C) to preheat and line a baking sheet with parchment paper.

2. In a mixing bowl, add two cups of shredded Cheddar cheese and two cups of shredded Parmesan cheese.

3. Add one teaspoon of garlic powder, one teaspoon of onion powder, 1/2 teaspoon of paprika, and 1/4 teaspoon of black pepper to the cheese mixture.

4. Mix the ingredients until well combined.

5. Take small spoonfuls of the cheese mixture and place them onto the prepared baking sheet, leaving enough space between each spoonful to allow for spreading.

6. Flatten each cheese mound slightly with the back of a spoon to form a thin, even layer.

7. Bake in the preheated oven for about 12-15 minutes or until the cheese crisps are golden brown and crispy.

8. Remove from the oven and let them cool on the baking sheet for a few minutes to allow them to firm up.

9. Carefully transfer the baked cheese crisps to a wire rack to cool completely. They will become even crispier as they cool.

10. Once completely cooled, store the cheese crisps in an airtight container. Enjoy as a low-fiber snack!

Nutritional Information (per serving):

- Carbs: 2g

- Fats: 28g

- Fiber: 0g

- Protein: 31g

Almond Butter and Banana Bites

Prep Time: 10 minutes
Cook Time: None (No cooking required)
Number of Servings: 4

Ingredients:

- 2 ripe bananas

- 1/2 cup almond butter

- 2 tablespoons honey

- 1/4 cup chopped almonds

- 1/4 cup shredded coconut

- 1/2 teaspoon vanilla extract

- Pinch of salt

Instructions:

1. Start by peeling and slicing 2 ripe bananas into bite-sized rounds, about 1/2 inch thick. Place half of the banana rounds on a parchment paper-lined tray.

2. In a small mixing bowl, add 1/2 cup of almond butter, two tablespoons of honey, 1/4 cup of chopped almonds, 1/4 cup of shredded coconut, 1/2 teaspoon of vanilla extract, and a pinch of salt. Mix until all the ingredients are well combined.

3. Take a spoonful of the almond butter mixture and place it on top of each banana round on the tray.

4. Top each almond butter-covered banana round with another banana round to create little "sandwiches."

5. Carefully press down to stick the banana rounds together, and the almond butter mixture will ooze out slightly to hold them in place.

6. Place the tray in the freezer for at least 2 hours or until the banana bites are firm and easy to handle.

7. Once frozen, transfer the almond butter and banana bites to an airtight container and store them in the freezer until you're ready to enjoy.

8. Serve these delightful low-fiber treats straight from the freezer and savor the combination of creamy almond butter and sweet banana!

Nutritional Information (per serving):

- Carbs: 18g

- Fats: 16g

- Fiber: 2g

- Protein: 6g

Spicy Roasted Edamame

Prep Time: 5 minutes
Cook Time: 20 minutes
Number of Servings: 4

Ingredients:

- 2 cups frozen edamame (unshelled)

- 1 tablespoon olive oil

- 1 teaspoon chili powder

- 1/2 teaspoon garlic powder

- 1/2 teaspoon onion powder

- 1/4 teaspoon cayenne pepper (adjust to taste)

- Salt, to taste

Instructions:

1. Turn on your oven and set it to 400°F (200°C) to preheat and line a baking sheet with parchment paper.

2. In a mixing bowl, add two cups of frozen edamame with one tablespoon of olive oil. Toss the edamame to coat them evenly with the oil.

3. In a separate small bowl, mix one teaspoon of chili powder, 1/2 teaspoon of garlic powder, 1/2 teaspoon of onion powder, and 1/4 teaspoon of cayenne pepper. Adjust the cayenne pepper to your desired level of spiciness.

4. Sprinkle the spice mixture over the oiled edamame and toss them again to ensure even coating.

5. Spread the seasoned edamame in a single layer on the prepared baking sheet.

6. Roast the edamame in the preheated oven for about 20 minutes, or until they become slightly crispy and golden, stirring them once or twice during cooking for even roasting.

7. Take out the spicy roasted edamame from the oven and immediately season with salt to taste while they're still hot.

8. Allow the edamame to cool for a few minutes before serving.

9. Enjoy these spicy roasted edamame as a delicious and low-fiber snack or appetizer!

Nutritional Information (per serving):

- Carbs: 6g

- Fats: 4g

- Fiber: 3g

- Protein: 8g

Coconut Yogurt with Mango

Prep Time: 10 minutes
Cook Time: None (No cooking required)
Number of Servings: 2

Ingredients:

- 2 cups unsweetened coconut yogurt
- 2 ripe mangoes, peeled, pitted, and diced
- 2 tablespoons honey (optional)
- 1/4 cup shredded coconut (optional)
- Fresh mint leaves for garnish (optional)

Instructions:

1. In a bowl, take two cups of unsweetened coconut yogurt.
2. Dice 2 ripe mangoes after peeling and removing the pits.
3. If you prefer a touch of sweetness, you can add two tablespoons of honey to the coconut yogurt. Mix sufficiently to combine. Note that this is optional, and you can adjust the sweetness to your preference.
4. Divide the diced mangoes into two serving bowls.
5. Spoon the sweetened or unsweetened coconut yogurt over the diced mangoes in each bowl.
6. Optionally, sprinkle 1/4 cup of shredded coconut over the yogurt and mango for extra flavor and texture.
7. Garnish with fresh mint leaves for a burst of color and freshness, if desired.
8. Serve the Coconut Yogurt with Mango immediately as a delightful and refreshing low-fiber dessert or breakfast.

Nutritional Information (per serving):

- Carbs: 42g
- Fats: 12g
- Fiber: 5g
- Protein: 2g

Smoked Salmon Cucumber Bites

Prep Time: 15 minutes
Cook Time: None (No cooking required)
Number of Servings: 4

Ingredients:

- 2 large cucumbers
- 4 ounces smoked salmon
- 1/2 cup cream cheese
- 2 tablespoons fresh dill, chopped
- 1 tablespoon capers, drained
- Freshly ground black pepper, to taste
- Lemon wedges for garnish (optional)

Instructions:

1. Begin by washing and drying 2 large cucumbers. Slice them into rounds, each about 1/4 inch thick. Set aside.

2. Take 4 ounces of smoked salmon and cut it into small pieces or strips. Set aside.

3. In a bowl, add 1/2 cup of cream cheese and two tablespoons of freshly chopped dill. Mix until the dill is evenly distributed throughout the cream cheese.

4. Drain one tablespoon of capers and set them aside.

5. To assemble each cucumber bite, spread a small amount of the dill cream cheese mixture onto a cucumber round.

6. Top the cream cheese with a piece of smoked salmon.

7. Place a caper on top of the smoked salmon.

8. Sprinkle a bit of freshly ground black pepper over the top for added flavor.

9. Optionally, garnish each bite with a lemon wedge for a refreshing citrus twist.

10. Repeat this process for the remaining cucumber rounds.

11. Arrange the Smoked Salmon Cucumber Bites on a serving platter.

12. Serve as an elegant and low-fiber appetizer or snack option.

Nutritional Information (per serving):

- Carbs: 5g

- Fats: 12g

- Fiber: 1g

- Protein: 6g

Herbed Tofu Cubes

Prep Time: 10 minutes
Cook Time: 15 minutes
Number of Servings: 4

Ingredients:

- 1 block (14 ounces) firm tofu

- 2 tablespoons olive oil

- 2 cloves garlic, minced

- 2 tablespoons fresh parsley, chopped

- 1 tablespoon fresh thyme leaves

- 1/2 teaspoon salt

- 1/4 teaspoon black pepper

- Zest of 1 lemon

- Juice of 1 lemon

Instructions:

1. Start by pressing the firm tofu to remove excess moisture. Place the tofu block between two paper towels or clean kitchen towels. Place a heavy object, such as a cast-iron skillet or a can of beans, on top of the tofu and let it sit for about 10 minutes. This will help the tofu firm up and absorb more flavor.

2. While the tofu is being pressed, chop two tablespoons of fresh parsley and measure out one tablespoon of fresh thyme leaves. Set them aside.

3. After the tofu has been pressed, cut it into 1-inch cubes.

4. In a bowl, add the cubed tofu with two tablespoons of olive oil, 2 cloves of minced garlic, the chopped parsley, thyme leaves, 1/2 teaspoon of salt, and 1/4 teaspoon of black pepper. Mix sufficiently to evenly coat the tofu with the herbs and seasonings.

5. Preheat a non-stick skillet over medium-high heat. Once hot, add the herbed tofu cubes to the skillet in a single layer.

6. Cook the tofu cubes for about 15 minutes, turning them occasionally, until golden brown and have a slightly crispy texture on the outside.

7. During the last few minutes of cooking, add the zest and juice of 1 lemon to the skillet. Stir to combine, allowing the lemon juice to coat the tofu cubes.

8. Once the Herbed Tofu Cubes are cooked to your liking, take them out from the heat.

9. Serve the tofu cubes as a delicious and low-fiber appetizer or as a protein-packed addition to salads or bowls.

Nutritional Information (per serving):

- Carbs: 5g

- Fats: 12g

- Fiber: 1g

- Protein: 9g

Pomegranate Seeds with Cottage Cheese

Prep Time: 10 minutes
Cook Time: None (No cooking required)
Number of Servings: 2

Ingredients:

- 1 cup cottage cheese

- 1/2 cup pomegranate seeds

- 1 tablespoon honey (optional)

- Fresh mint leaves for garnish (optional)

Instructions:

1. Begin by measuring one cup of cottage cheese.

2. Take 1/2 cup of fresh pomegranate seeds. You can buy pre-packaged pomegranate seeds or extract them from a fresh pomegranate.

3. Optionally, for added sweetness, drizzle one tablespoon of honey over the cottage cheese. This step is entirely optional, and you can adjust the sweetness to your liking.

4. Gently fold the pomegranate seeds into the cottage cheese, ensuring evenly distributed.

5. If desired, garnish the Pomegranate Seeds with Cottage Cheese with fresh mint leaves for a burst of color and freshness.

6. Serve immediately as a light and low-fiber dessert, breakfast, or snack.

Nutritional Information (per serving):

- Carbs: 17g

- Fats: 4g

- Fiber: 2g

- Protein: 14g

Cinnamon Almonds

Prep Time: 5 minutes
Cook Time: 15 minutes
Number of Servings: 4

Ingredients:

- 2 cups whole almonds

- 1/4 cup granulated sugar

- 1/2 teaspoon ground cinnamon

- 1/4 teaspoon salt

- 1/4 cup water

- 1/2 teaspoon vanilla extract

Instructions:

1. Turn on your oven and set it to 350°F (175°C) to preheat and line a baking sheet with parchment paper.

2. In a mixing bowl, add two cups of whole almonds, 1/4 cup of granulated sugar, 1/2 teaspoon of ground cinnamon, and 1/4 teaspoon of salt. Mix sufficiently to evenly coat the almonds with the sugar and spices.

3. In a saucepan, add 1/4 cup of water and 1/2 teaspoon of vanilla extract. Heat over medium-high heat until it starts to simmer.

4. Add the sugar-coated almonds to the simmering water and stir constantly. The water will gradually evaporate, leaving behind a sticky syrup that coats the almonds.

5. Continue stirring and cooking for about 5-7 minutes until the syrup thickens and coats the almonds in a glossy layer.

6. Quickly transfer the glazed almonds to the prepared baking sheet, spreading them out in a single layer to prevent them from sticking together.

7. Place the baking sheet in the preheated oven and bake for about 10 minutes, or until the almonds are golden brown and fragrant. Keep an eye on them to avoid burning.

8. Take out the Cinnamon Almonds from the oven and let them cool completely on the baking sheet. As they cool, the sugar coating will harden.

9. Once cooled, break the almonds apart and store them in an airtight container.

10. Enjoy these sweet and fragrant Cinnamon Almonds as a delightful and low-fiber snack!

Nutritional Information (per serving):

- Carbs: 14g

- Fats: 18g

- Fiber: 3g

- Protein: 6g

Guacamole with Jicama Sticks

Prep Time: 15 minutes
Cook Time: None (No cooking required)
Number of Servings: 4

Ingredients:

- 3 ripe avocados

- 1 small red onion, finely diced

- 2 tomatoes, diced

- 2 cloves garlic, minced

- Juice of 2 limes

- 1/4 cup fresh cilantro, chopped

- Salt and black pepper, to taste

- 1 large jicama, peeled and cut into sticks for dipping

Instructions:

1. Start by cutting the avocados in half, removing the pits, and scooping the flesh into a mixing bowl.

2. Mash the avocados using a fork or potato masher until you achieve your desired level of guacamole chunkiness.

3. Finely dice 1 small red onion and add it to the mashed avocados.

4. Dice 2 tomatoes and add them to the mixing bowl.

5. Mince 2 cloves of garlic and add them to the mixture.

6. Squeeze the juice of 2 limes into the bowl to give the guacamole a tangy kick.

7. Chop 1/4 cup of fresh cilantro and add it to the guacamole for a burst of flavor.

8. Season the guacamole with salt and black pepper to taste. Mix all the ingredients together until well combined.

9. Peel a large jicama and cut it into sticks for dipping. You can also use other vegetables or tortilla chips as dippers if you prefer.

10. Serve the Guacamole with Jicama Sticks as a tasty and low-fiber snack, appetizer, or party dip.

Nutritional Information (per serving):

- Carbs: 17g

- Fats: 15g

- Fiber: 9g

- Protein: 3g

Baked Pears with Cinnamon

Prep Time: 10 minutes
Cook Time: 30 minutes
Number of Servings: 4

Ingredients:

- 4 ripe but firm pears

- 2 tablespoons unsalted butter

- 2 tablespoons honey

- 1/2 teaspoon ground cinnamon

- 1/4 teaspoon vanilla extract

- A pinch of salt

- Vanilla ice cream or yogurt for serving (optional)

Instructions:

1. Turn on your oven and set it to 375°F (190°C) to preheat and line a baking dish with parchment paper.

2. Wash and dry 4 ripe but firm pears. Leave the skins on, but you can core them if desired.

3. In a microwave-safe bowl, melt two tablespoons of unsalted butter in the microwave.

4. Add two tablespoons of honey to the melted butter and stir to combine.

5. Mix in 1/2 teaspoon of ground cinnamon, 1/4 teaspoon of vanilla extract, and a pinch of salt. Stir until the mixture is well blended.

6. Place the prepared pears in the lined baking dish.

7. Drizzle the honey-butter mixture evenly over the pears, ensuring each pear is coated.

8. Bake the pears in the preheated oven for about 30 minutes or until tender and easily pierced with a fork. Baking time may vary depending on the size and ripeness of the pears.

9. While baking, baste the pears with the syrup in the baking dish a couple of times to ensure evenly coated and caramelized.

10. Take out the Baked Pears with Cinnamon from the oven and let them cool slightly.

11. Serve the baked pears warm, optionally with a scoop of vanilla ice cream or a dollop of yogurt if desired.

12. Enjoy this delightful and low-fiber dessert!

Nutritional Information (per serving, without optional toppings):

- Carbs: 34g

- Fats: 6g

- Fiber: 5g

- Protein: 1g

Rice Cakes with Peanut Butter

Prep Time: 5 minutes
Cook Time: None (No cooking required)
Number of Servings: 2

Ingredients:

- 4 rice cakes

- 4 tablespoons natural peanut butter

- 1 small banana, sliced

- 1 tablespoon honey (optional)
- A pinch of salt

Instructions:

1. Start by laying out 4 rice cakes on a clean surface.
2. Measure out 4 tablespoons of natural peanut butter.
3. Spread a generous layer of peanut butter onto each rice cake.
4. Slice 1 small banana into thin rounds.
5. Place the banana slices on top of the peanut butter-covered rice cakes.
6. If desired, drizzle one tablespoon of honey over the banana-topped rice cakes. This step is optional and can be adjusted to your preferred level of sweetness.
7. Finish with a pinch of salt over the top to enhance the flavors.
8. Your Rice Cakes with Peanut Butter are ready to be enjoyed as a quick and satisfying low-fiber snack or light meal.

Nutritional Information (per serving):

- Carbs: 39g
- Fats: 19g
- Fiber: 3g
- Protein: 11g

Baked Potato Chips

Prep Time: 10 minutes
Cook Time: 20 minutes
Number of Servings: 4

Ingredients:

- 4 medium russet potatoes
- 2 tablespoons olive oil
- 1/2 teaspoon paprika

- 1/2 teaspoon garlic powder

- 1/2 teaspoon onion powder

- 1/4 teaspoon salt

- 1/4 teaspoon black pepper

Instructions:

1. Turn on your oven and set it to 425°F (220°C) to preheat and line two baking sheets with parchment paper.

2. Wash and scrub 4 medium russet potatoes thoroughly to remove any dirt or debris.

3. Using a sharp knife or a mandoline slicer, slice the potatoes into thin rounds, about 1/8 inch thick.

4. In a large mixing bowl, add the potato slices with two tablespoons of olive oil. Toss to ensure the potato slices are evenly coated with the oil.

5. In a separate small bowl, mix 1/2 teaspoon of paprika, 1/2 teaspoon of garlic powder, 1/2 teaspoon of onion powder, 1/4 teaspoon of salt, and 1/4 teaspoon of black pepper.

6. Sprinkle the spice mixture over the oiled potato slices and toss again to evenly distribute the spices.

7. Arrange the seasoned potato slices in a single layer on the prepared baking sheets, ensuring they do not overlap.

8. Place the baking sheets in the preheated oven and bake for about 15-20 minutes, flipping the potato slices halfway through the baking time, until the chips are golden brown and crispy.

9. Keep a close eye on them to prevent burning, as the cooking time may vary based on the thickness of your slices.

10. Once the Baked Potato Chips are done, take them out from the oven and let them cool on the baking sheets for a few minutes. They will become even crispier as they cool.

11. Transfer the baked chips to a serving platter and enjoy your homemade, low-fiber potato chips as a healthier snack option!

Nutritional Information (per serving):

- Carbs: 34g

- Fats: 7g

- Fiber: 2g

- Protein: 3g

Greek Yogurt with Honey

Prep Time: 5 minutes
Cook Time: None (No cooking required)
Number of Servings: 2

Ingredients:

- 2 cups plain Greek yogurt

- 4 tablespoons honey (adjust to taste)

Instructions:

1. Start by measuring out two cups of plain Greek yogurt.

2. In a bowl, spoon 4 tablespoons of honey. You can adjust the amount of honey to your preferred level of sweetness.

3. Drizzle the honey over the Greek yogurt.

4. Using a spoon or a whisk, gently swirl the honey into the yogurt, ensuring it's evenly distributed.

5. Continue to swirl until the honey is fully incorporated with the yogurt, creating a sweet and creamy mixture.

6. Serve the Greek Yogurt with Honey in individual bowls or glasses.

7. Enjoy this simple and low-fiber dessert or snack that's both delicious and nutritious!

Nutritional Information (per serving):

- Carbs: 36g

- Fats: 0g

- Fiber: 0g

- Protein: 22g

Cottage Cheese and Pineapple

Prep Time: 5 minutes
Cook Time: None (No cooking required)
Number of Servings: 2

Ingredients:

- 1 cup low-fat cottage cheese
- 1 cup diced pineapple (fresh or canned, drained)
- 1 tablespoon honey (optional)

Instructions:

1. Begin by measuring out one cup of low-fat cottage cheese.

2. Dice one cup of pineapple. You can use either fresh or canned pineapple, but if using canned, be sure to drain the pineapple pieces.

3. Optionally, for added sweetness, drizzle one tablespoon of honey over the cottage cheese and pineapple. This step is entirely optional, and you can adjust the sweetness to your preference.

4. Gently stir the honey into the mixture to evenly distribute the sweetness.

5. Serve the Cottage Cheese and Pineapple in individual bowls or glasses.

6. Enjoy this simple and nutritious low-fiber snack or dessert!

Nutritional Information (per serving, without optional honey):

- Carbs: 26g
- Fats: 2g
- Fiber: 2g
- Protein: 20g

Apple Slices with Almond Butter

Prep Time: 5 minutes
Cook Time: None (No cooking required)
Number of Servings: 2

Ingredients:

- 2 medium apples (any variety)
- 4 tablespoons almond butter

Instructions:

1. Begin by washing and drying 2 medium apples. You can use any apple variety you prefer.
2. Core the apples and slice them into thin rounds or wedges.
3. Measure out 4 tablespoons of almond butter.
4. To serve, spread almond butter on the apple slices or use it as a dip for the apple slices.
5. Arrange the Apple Slices with Almond Butter on a plate or platter.
6. Enjoy this quick and nutritious low-fiber snack!

Nutritional Information (per serving):

- Carbs: 26g
- Fats: 16g
- Fiber: 4g
- Protein: 6g

Trail Mix with Nuts and Dried Fruit

Prep Time: 5 minutes
Cook Time: None (No cooking required)
Number of Servings: 4

Ingredients:

- 1 cup mixed nuts (almonds, cashews, and peanuts)
- 1/2 cup dried cranberries
- 1/2 cup raisins
- 1/4 cup dark chocolate chips
- 1/4 cup banana chips (optional)
- 1/4 cup pumpkin seeds (pepitas)

Instructions:

1. In a large bowl, add one cup of mixed nuts. You can use a variety of nuts like almonds, cashews, and peanuts.

2. Add 1/2 cup of dried cranberries to the nuts in the bowl.

3. Measure out 1/2 cup of raisins and add them to the mix.

4. Toss in 1/4 cup of dark chocolate chips. You can adjust the amount to your taste.

5. Optionally, include 1/4 cup of banana chips for extra flavor and texture.

6. Complete the mix with 1/4 cup of pumpkin seeds (pepitas).

7. Gently stir all the ingredients together to ensure an even distribution of nuts, dried fruits, seeds, and chocolate chips.

8. Your Trail Mix with Nuts and Dried Fruit is ready to be enjoyed as a delicious and convenient low-fiber snack for on-the-go or anytime!

Nutritional Information (per serving):

- Carbs: 38g
- Fats: 21g
- Fiber: 3g
- Protein: 9g

Baked Sweet Potato Fries

Prep Time: 15 minutes
Cook Time: 30 minutes
Number of Servings: 4

Ingredients:

- 4 medium sweet potatoes
- 2 tablespoons olive oil
- 1 teaspoon paprika
- 1/2 teaspoon garlic powder

- 1/2 teaspoon onion powder
- 1/2 teaspoon salt
- 1/4 teaspoon black pepper

Instructions:

1. Turn on your oven and set it to 425°F (220°C) to preheat and line a baking sheet with parchment paper.

2. Wash and peel 4 medium sweet potatoes.

3. Slice the sweet potatoes into thin strips, similar to the size and shape of traditional French fries.

4. In a large mixing bowl, add the sweet potato strips with two tablespoons of olive oil. Toss to ensure the sweet potato strips are evenly coated with the oil.

5. In a separate small bowl, mix one teaspoon of paprika, 1/2 teaspoon of garlic powder, 1/2 teaspoon of onion powder, 1/2 teaspoon of salt, and 1/4 teaspoon of black pepper.

6. Sprinkle the spice mixture over the oiled sweet potato strips and toss again to evenly distribute the spices.

7. Arrange the seasoned sweet potato strips on the prepared baking sheet, ensuring spread out in a single layer to allow for even cooking.

8. Place the baking sheet in the preheated oven and bake for about 25-30 minutes, flipping the sweet potato fries halfway through the baking time, until golden brown and crispy.

9. Keep a close eye on them to prevent burning, as the cooking time may vary based on the thickness of your sweet potato fries.

10. Once the Baked Sweet Potato Fries are done, take them out from the oven and let them cool slightly.

11. Serve the sweet potato fries as a delicious and healthier alternative to traditional fries. Enjoy!

Nutritional Information (per serving):

- Carbs: 30g
- Fats: 6g

- Fiber: 4g

- Protein: 2g

Roasted Chickpeas

Prep Time: 10 minutes
Cook Time: 30 minutes
Number of Servings: 4

Ingredients:

- 2 cans (15 ounces each) canned chickpeas (garbanzo beans)

- 2 tablespoons olive oil

- 1 teaspoon paprika

- 1/2 teaspoon ground cumin

- 1/2 teaspoon garlic powder

- 1/2 teaspoon onion powder

- 1/2 teaspoon salt

- 1/4 teaspoon black pepper

Instructions:

1. Turn on your oven and set it to 400°F (200°C) to preheat and line a baking sheet with parchment paper.

2. Open and drain 2 cans (15 ounces each) of canned chickpeas (garbanzo beans). Rinse them thoroughly under cold water and pat them dry with paper towels.

3. In a large mixing bowl, add the dried chickpeas with two tablespoons of olive oil. Toss to ensure the chickpeas are evenly coated with the oil.

4. In a separate small bowl, mix one teaspoon of paprika, 1/2 teaspoon of ground cumin, 1/2 teaspoon of garlic powder, 1/2 teaspoon of onion powder, 1/2 teaspoon of salt, and 1/4 teaspoon of black pepper.

5. Sprinkle the spice mixture over the oiled chickpeas and toss again to evenly distribute the spices.

6. Spread the seasoned chickpeas in a single layer on the prepared baking sheet.

7. Place the baking sheet in the preheated oven and roast the chickpeas for about 30 minutes, or until golden brown and crunchy. Shake the pan or stir the chickpeas occasionally for even cooking.

8. Keep an eye on them towards the end of the cooking time to prevent over-browning.

9. Once the Roasted Chickpeas are done, take them out from the oven and let them cool on the baking sheet.

10. Serve the roasted chickpeas as a tasty and nutritious low-fiber snack or as a crunchy topping for salads and bowls.

Nutritional Information (per serving):

- Carbs: 20g

- Fats: 6g

- Fiber: 5g

- Protein: 6g

Hummus with Carrot Sticks

Prep Time: 10 minutes
Cook Time: None (No cooking required)
Number of Servings: 4

Ingredients:

- 2 cups canned chickpeas (garbanzo beans), drained and rinsed

- 1/4 cup tahini

- 2 cloves garlic, minced

- Juice of 1 lemon

- 2 tablespoons olive oil

- 1/2 teaspoon ground cumin

- Salt, to taste

- Black pepper, to taste
- 4 large carrots, peeled and cut into sticks for dipping

Instructions:

1. In a food processor, add two cups of canned chickpeas (garbanzo beans), drained and rinsed.

2. Add 1/4 cup of tahini to the chickpeas in the food processor.

3. Mince 2 cloves of garlic and add them to the mix.

4. Squeeze the juice of 1 lemon into the food processor for a tangy kick.

5. Pour in two tablespoons of olive oil.

6. Sprinkle in 1/2 teaspoon of ground cumin for added flavor.

7. Season the mixture with salt and black pepper to taste.

8. Blend all the ingredients in the food processor until you achieve a smooth and creamy hummus consistency. You may need to scrape down the sides of the bowl and blend again to ensure everything is well combined.

9. Once the hummus is ready, transfer it to a serving bowl.

10. Prepare 4 large carrots by peeling them and cutting them into sticks for dipping.

11. Serve the Hummus with Carrot Sticks as a nutritious and low-fiber snack or appetizer.

Nutritional Information (per serving):

- Carbs: 22g
- Fats: 15g
- Fiber: 6g
- Protein: 9g

Cheese and Crackers

Prep Time: 5 minutes
Cook Time: None (No cooking required)
Number of Servings: 4

Ingredients:

- 8 ounces of your favorite cheese (Cheddar, Swiss, etc.), sliced
- 1 sleeve (about 40) whole-grain crackers

Instructions:

1. Start by arranging 8 ounces of your favorite cheese on a serving platter. You can use Cheddar, Swiss, or any cheese of your choice. Slice the cheese for easy serving.

2. Next, place 1 sleeve (about 40) of whole-grain crackers on the same platter or on a separate one.

3. Serve the Cheese and Crackers as a simple and tasty low-fiber snack or appetizer.

4. Enjoy the combination of creamy cheese and crunchy crackers!

Nutritional Information (per serving):

- Carbs: 15g
- Fats: 21g
- Fiber: 2g
- Protein: 14g

DESSERTS

Raspberry Chia Seed Pudding

Prep Time: 10 minutes
Cook Time: 0 minutes
Number of Servings: 2

Ingredients:

- 1 cup fresh raspberries
- 2 cups unsweetened almond milk
- 1/2 cup chia seeds
- 2 tablespoons honey
- 1 teaspoon vanilla extract

Instructions:

1. In a blender, add 1/2 cup of fresh raspberries, one cup of unsweetened almond milk, and one tablespoon of honey. Blend until smooth.

2. In a mixing bowl, add two cups of unsweetened almond milk, 1/2 cup of chia seeds, one tablespoon of honey, and one teaspoon of vanilla extract. Mix sufficiently.

3. Pour the raspberry almond milk mixture from the blender into the chia seed mixture. Stir until all ingredients are well combined.

4. Cover the bowl and refrigerate for at least 4 hours or overnight to allow the chia seeds to absorb the liquid and thicken the pudding.

5. Before serving, divide the raspberry chia seed pudding into two serving glasses or bowls.

6. Top each serving with the remaining fresh raspberries.

Nutritional Information (per serving):

- Carbs: 28 grams
- Fats: 15 grams
- Fiber: 14 grams
- Protein: 6 grams

Lemon Sorbet with Basil

Prep Time: 10 minutes
Cook Time: 0 minutes
Number of Servings: 4

Ingredients:

- 1 cup freshly squeezed lemon juice

- 1 cup water

- 1 cup granulated sugar

- 2 tablespoons fresh basil leaves, finely chopped

- Zest of 1 lemon

Instructions:

1. In a saucepan, add one cup of water and one cup of granulated sugar. Heat over medium heat, stirring until the sugar completely dissolves. This will create a simple syrup. Allow it to cool.

2. Once the simple syrup has cooled, add one cup of freshly squeezed lemon juice and the zest of 1 lemon to the syrup. Mix sufficiently.

3. Transfer the lemon mixture to an ice cream maker and churn according to the manufacturer's instructions. This typically takes about 20-25 minutes.

4. During the last few minutes of churning, add two tablespoons of finely chopped fresh basil leaves to the sorbet mixture. Let it incorporate evenly.

5. Once the sorbet has reached a firm, ice-cream-like consistency, transfer it to an airtight container and freeze for an extra 2 hours to firm up further.

6. Before serving, allow the sorbet to sit at room temperature for a few minutes to soften slightly, making it easier to scoop.

Nutritional Information (per serving):

- Carbs: 42 grams

- Fats: 0 grams

- Fiber: 0 grams

- Protein: 0 grams

Chocolate Avocado Mousse

Prep Time: 10 minutes
Cook Time: 0 minutes
Number of Servings: 4

Ingredients:

- 2 ripe avocados, peeled and pitted

- 1/2 cup unsweetened cocoa powder

- 1/4 cup honey or maple syrup

- 1/4 cup unsweetened almond milk

- 1 teaspoon vanilla extract

- A pinch of salt

- Optional toppings: whipped cream, shaved chocolate, or fresh berries

Instructions:

1. In a food processor or blender, add 2 ripe avocados, 1/2 cup of unsweetened cocoa powder, 1/4 cup of honey or maple syrup, 1/4 cup of unsweetened almond milk, one teaspoon of vanilla extract, and a pinch of salt.

2. Blend the ingredients until smooth and creamy, scraping down the sides of the bowl as needed to ensure everything is well combined. You should have a rich, chocolatey mousse-like texture.

3. Taste the mousse and adjust the sweetness if needed by adding more honey or maple syrup and blend again until well incorporated.

4. Divide the chocolate avocado mousse into 4 serving glasses or bowls.

5. If desired, top each serving with a dollop of whipped cream, some shaved chocolate, or fresh berries.

6. Refrigerate for at least 30 minutes before serving to allow the mousse to chill and set slightly.

Nutritional Information (per serving):

- Carbs: 23 grams

- Fats: 14 grams

- Fiber: 8 grams

- Protein: 3 grams

Baked Peaches with Cinnamon

Prep Time: 10 minutes
Cook Time: 25 minutes
Number of Servings: 4

Ingredients:

- 4 ripe peaches, halved and pitted

- 2 tablespoons unsalted butter, melted

- 2 tablespoons honey

- 1 teaspoon ground cinnamon

- 1/4 teaspoon vanilla extract

- A pinch of salt

- Vanilla ice cream or whipped cream for serving (optional)

Instructions:

1. Turn on your oven and set it to 375°F (190°C) to preheat.

2. In a small bowl, add two tablespoons of melted unsalted butter, two tablespoons of honey, one teaspoon of ground cinnamon, 1/4 teaspoon of vanilla extract, and a pinch of salt. Mix sufficiently to create the cinnamon honey butter.

3. Place the halved and pitted peaches, cut side up, on a baking sheet or in a baking dish.

4. Brush the peaches generously with the cinnamon honey butter mixture, ensuring well coated.

5. Bake the peaches in the preheated oven for about 25 minutes or until tender and slightly caramelized.

6. Take out the baked peaches from the oven and let them cool slightly before serving.

7. If desired, serve the baked peaches with a scoop of vanilla ice cream or a dollop of whipped cream for an extra treat.

Nutritional Information (per serving, without optional toppings):

- Carbs: 21 grams

- Fats: 6 grams

- Fiber: 2 grams

- Protein: 1 gram

Coconut Flour Banana Bread

Prep Time: 10 minutes
Cook Time: 45 minutes
Number of Servings: 8

Ingredients:

- 4 ripe bananas, mashed

- 4 large eggs

- 1/2 cup coconut flour

- 1/4 cup melted coconut oil

- 1/4 cup honey or maple syrup

- 1 teaspoon baking powder

- 1 teaspoon vanilla extract

- 1/2 teaspoon ground cinnamon

- A pinch of salt

Instructions:

1. Turn on your oven and set it to 350°F (175°C) to preheat. Grease a 9x5-inch (23x13 cm) loaf pan and line it with parchment paper for easy removal.

2. In a mixing bowl, add the mashed bananas, 4 large eggs, 1/2 cup of coconut flour, 1/4 cup of melted coconut oil, 1/4 cup of honey or maple syrup, one teaspoon of baking powder, one teaspoon of vanilla extract, 1/2 teaspoon of ground cinnamon, and a pinch of salt.

3. Mix the ingredients together until a smooth batter forms. Ensure there are no lumps in the batter.

4. Pour the banana bread batter into the prepared loaf pan.

5. Bake in the preheated oven for about 45 minutes or until a toothpick inserted into the center comes out clean and the top is golden brown.

6. Take out the banana bread from the oven and allow it to cool in the pan for 10-15 minutes.

7. After cooling in the pan, transfer the banana bread to a wire rack to cool completely.

8. Once cooled, slice and serve.

Nutritional Information (per serving):

- Carbs: 17 grams

- Fats: 10 grams

- Fiber: 4 grams

- Protein: 4 grams

Almond Flour Shortbread Cookies

Prep Time: 15 minutes
Cook Time: 12 minutes
Number of Servings: 12 cookies

Ingredients:

- 1 1/2 cups almond flour

- 1/4 cup unsalted butter, softened

- 1/4 cup powdered erythritol or your preferred low-carb sweetener

- 1 teaspoon vanilla extract

- 1/4 teaspoon salt

Instructions:

1. Turn on your oven and set it to 350°F (175°C) to preheat. Line a baking sheet with parchment paper.

2. In a mixing bowl, add 1 1/2 cups of almond flour, 1/4 cup of softened unsalted butter, 1/4 cup of powdered erythritol (or your preferred low-carb sweetener), one teaspoon of vanilla extract, and 1/4 teaspoon of salt.

3. Mix the ingredients together until a crumbly dough forms. You can use your hands to knead the dough gently to ensure it comes together.

4. Form the dough into a ball and place it between two sheets of parchment paper.

5. Roll out the dough to about 1/4-inch (0.6 cm) thickness.

6. Use cookie cutters to cut out desired shapes from the dough. Place the cut-out cookies onto the prepared baking sheet.

7. Gather any remaining dough scraps, roll them out again, and continue to cut out cookies until all the dough is used.

8. Bake the cookies in the preheated oven for about 10-12 minutes or until the edges are lightly golden.

9. Take out the cookies from the oven and let them cool on the baking sheet for a few minutes before transferring them to a wire rack to cool completely.

10. Once cooled, the almond flour shortbread cookies are ready to enjoy.

Nutritional Information (per cookie):

- Carbs: 2 grams

- Fats: 8 grams

- Fiber: 1 gram

- Protein: 2 grams

Vanilla Panna Cotta

Prep Time: 10 minutes
Cook Time: 10 minutes
Chill Time: 4 hours
Number of Servings: 4

Ingredients:

- 1 cup heavy cream
- 1 cup whole milk
- 1/2 cup granulated sugar
- 1 vanilla bean or one teaspoon pure vanilla extract
- 2 1/2 teaspoons unflavored gelatin
- 2 tablespoons cold water

Instructions:

1. Pour two tablespoons of cold water into a small bowl and sprinkle 2 1/2 teaspoons of unflavored gelatin evenly over the water. Let it sit for about 5 minutes to allow the gelatin to bloom.

2. If using a vanilla bean, split it in half lengthwise and scrape out the seeds with the back of a knife. In a saucepan, add the seeds (or one teaspoon of pure vanilla extract), one cup of heavy cream, one cup of whole milk, and 1/2 cup of granulated sugar.

3. Heat the mixture over medium-low heat, stirring constantly until it's hot but not boiling. Remove it from the heat.

4. If you used a vanilla bean, take out the bean pod at this point.

5. Microwave the bloomed gelatin for about 10-15 seconds until it's completely melted.

6. Stir the melted gelatin into the milk and cream mixture until well combined.

7. Pour the mixture evenly into 4 serving glasses or ramekins.

8. Allow the panna cotta to cool at room temperature for about 15-20 minutes, then cover each glass with plastic wrap and refrigerate for at least 4 hours or until set.

9. Before serving, you can garnish with fresh berries, fruit compote, or a drizzle of caramel if desired.

Nutritional Information (per serving):

- Carbs: 21 grams

- Fats: 29 grams

- Fiber: 0 grams

- Protein: 4 grams

Pecan Pralines

Prep Time: 10 minutes
Cook Time: 10 minutes
Number of Servings: 16

Ingredients:

- 1 cup granulated sugar

- 1 cup packed light brown sugar

- 1/2 cup heavy cream

- 4 tablespoons unsalted butter

- 2 cups pecan halves

- 1 teaspoon pure vanilla extract

- 1/4 teaspoon salt

Instructions:

1. Line a baking sheet with parchment paper or a silicone baking mat and set it aside.

2. In a heavy-bottomed saucepan, add one cup of granulated sugar, one cup of packed light brown sugar, 1/2 cup of heavy cream, and 4 tablespoons of unsalted butter.

3. Cook over medium heat, stirring constantly, until the mixture comes to a boil. Once it boils, insert a candy thermometer into the mixture.

4. Keep on cooking the mixture, stirring frequently, until it reaches the "soft-ball" stage on the candy thermometer, which is about

236°F (113°C) to preheat. This should take approximately 5-7 minutes.

5. Once the mixture reaches the soft-ball stage, remove it from the heat and quickly stir in two cups of pecan halves, one teaspoon of pure vanilla extract, and 1/4 teaspoon of salt. Stir until the pecans are well coated.

6. Working quickly, use a spoon to drop spoonfuls of the praline mixture onto the prepared baking sheet. If the mixture starts to harden in the saucepan, you can gently reheat it over low heat.

7. Allow the pecan pralines to cool and harden at room temperature for about 30 minutes to 1 hour.

8. Once completely set and firm, carefully take out the pralines from the parchment paper and store them in an airtight container.

Nutritional Information (per serving):

- Carbs: 25 grams

- Fats: 13 grams

- Fiber: 1 gram

- Protein: 1 gram

Cocoa-Dusted Truffles

Prep Time: 20 minutes
Chill Time: 2 hours
Number of Servings: 20 truffles

Ingredients:

- 8 ounces (1 1/2 cups) semisweet chocolate chips

- 1/2 cup heavy cream

- 2 tablespoons unsalted butter

- 1 teaspoon pure vanilla extract

- 1/4 teaspoon salt

- 1/4 cup unsweetened cocoa powder, for dusting

Instructions:

1. In a microwave-safe bowl or a heatproof bowl set over a pot of simmering water (double boiler), add 8 ounces (1 1/2 cups) of semisweet chocolate chips and 1/2 cup of heavy cream.

2. Heat the mixture in the microwave in 20-30 second intervals, stirring after each interval until the chocolate is completely melted and the mixture is smooth. If using a double boiler, stir until the chocolate is melted and smooth.

3. Stir in two tablespoons of unsalted butter until fully incorporated into the chocolate mixture.

4. Add one teaspoon of pure vanilla extract and 1/4 teaspoon of salt to the chocolate mixture. Stir until well combined.

5. Pour the chocolate mixture into a shallow dish or a baking pan lined with parchment paper. Spread it out evenly.

6. Refrigerate the mixture for at least 2 hours or until it is firm and easy to handle.

7. Once the mixture is firm, use a spoon or a melon baller to scoop out small portions and roll them into 1-inch (2.5 cm) truffle balls.

8. Place 1/4 cup of unsweetened cocoa powder in a shallow bowl.

9. Roll each truffle in the cocoa powder, coating them evenly. Shake off any excess cocoa powder.

10. Arrange the cocoa-dusted truffles on a serving platter or in mini paper candy cups.

11. Store the truffles in an airtight container in the refrigerator until ready to serve.

Nutritional Information (per truffle):

- Carbs: 6 grams
- Fats: 6 grams
- Fiber: 1 gram
- Protein: 1 gram

Cardamom Rice Pudding

Prep Time: 10 minutes
Cook Time: 40 minutes
Number of Servings: 4

Ingredients:

- 1/2 cup long-grain white rice
- 4 cups whole milk
- 1/2 cup granulated sugar
- 1 teaspoon ground cardamom
- 1/2 teaspoon pure vanilla extract
- A pinch of salt
- Slivered almonds and ground cinnamon for garnish (optional)

Instructions:

1. Rinse 1/2 cup of long-grain white rice under cold water until the water runs clear. Drain well.

2. In a large saucepan, add the rinsed rice, 4 cups of whole milk, and a pinch of salt. Place the saucepan over medium-high heat and bring the mixture to a boil.

3. Once the mixture boils, reduce the heat to low and let it simmer, uncovered, for about 30-35 minutes, or until the rice is tender and the mixture thickens, stirring occasionally.

4. Stir in 1/2 cup of granulated sugar, one teaspoon of ground cardamom, and 1/2 teaspoon of pure vanilla extract. Continue to simmer for an extra 5 minutes, stirring constantly until the sugar is fully dissolved and the flavors meld.

5. Take out the cardamom rice pudding from the heat and let it cool slightly.

6. If desired, garnish the pudding with slivered almonds and a sprinkle of ground cinnamon.

7. Serve the rice pudding warm or chilled, as you prefer.

Nutritional Information (per serving):

- Carbs: 54 grams

- Fats: 10 grams

- Fiber: 0 grams

- Protein: 9 grams

Chocolate Avocado Pudding

Prep Time: 10 minutes
Chill Time: 1 hour
Number of Servings: 4

Ingredients:

- 2 ripe avocados, peeled and pitted

- 1/2 cup unsweetened cocoa powder

- 1/4 cup honey or maple syrup

- 1/4 cup unsweetened almond milk

- 1 teaspoon pure vanilla extract

- A pinch of salt

Instructions:

1. In a food processor or blender, add 2 ripe avocados, 1/2 cup of unsweetened cocoa powder, 1/4 cup of honey or maple syrup, 1/4 cup of unsweetened almond milk, one teaspoon of pure vanilla extract, and a pinch of salt.

2. Blend the ingredients until you have a smooth and creamy pudding-like consistency. Make sure there are no lumps.

3. Taste the chocolate avocado pudding and adjust the sweetness if needed by adding more honey or maple syrup, and blend again until well incorporated.

4. Transfer the pudding into serving glasses or bowls.

5. Cover the glasses or bowls with plastic wrap, ensuring that the plastic wrap touches the surface of the pudding to prevent it from forming a skin.

6. Refrigerate the pudding for at least 1 hour to chill and set.

7. Before serving, you can garnish the chocolate avocado pudding with fresh berries, whipped cream, or a dusting of cocoa powder if desired.

Nutritional Information (per serving):

- Carbs: 29 grams

- Fats: 13 grams

- Fiber: 9 grams

- Protein: 3 grams

Rice Pudding

Prep Time: 10 minutes
Cook Time: 25 minutes
Chill Time: 2 hours
Number of Servings: 6

Ingredients:

- 1 cup white rice

- 4 cups whole milk

- 1/2 cup granulated sugar

- 1 teaspoon pure vanilla extract

- 1/4 teaspoon ground cinnamon

- 1/4 teaspoon salt

- Optional toppings: ground cinnamon, raisins, or a sprinkle of nutmeg

Instructions:

1. Rinse one cup of white rice under cold water until the water runs clear. Drain well.

2. In a large saucepan, add the rinsed rice and 4 cups of whole milk. Place the saucepan over medium-high heat and bring the mixture to a boil.

3. Once the mixture boils, reduce the heat to low and let it simmer, uncovered, for about 15-20 minutes, or until the rice is tender and the mixture thickens, stirring frequently.

4. Stir in 1/2 cup of granulated sugar, one teaspoon of pure vanilla extract, 1/4 teaspoon of ground cinnamon, and 1/4 teaspoon of salt. Continue to simmer for an extra 5 minutes, stirring constantly until the sugar is fully dissolved and the flavors meld.

5. Take out the rice pudding from the heat and let it cool slightly.

6. If desired, you can sprinkle some ground cinnamon, add raisins, or a touch of nutmeg as toppings.

7. Transfer the rice pudding to a serving dish or individual serving bowls.

8. Cover with plastic wrap, ensuring that the plastic wrap touches the surface of the pudding to prevent it from forming a skin.

9. Refrigerate the rice pudding for at least 2 hours to chill and set.

10. Serve the rice pudding chilled, either as is or with your preferred toppings.

Nutritional Information (per serving, without optional toppings):

- Carbs: 51 grams
- Fats: 8 grams
- Fiber: 0 grams
- Protein: 8 grams

Lemon Sorbet

Prep Time: 15 minutes
Chill Time: 3 hours
Number of Servings: 6

Ingredients:

- 1 cup freshly squeezed lemon juice (about 6-8 lemons)
- 1 cup water
- 1 cup granulated sugar

- Zest of 2 lemons

- A pinch of salt

- Lemon slices and fresh mint leaves for garnish (optional)

Instructions:

1. In a saucepan, add one cup of water and one cup of granulated sugar. Heat over medium heat, stirring until the sugar completely dissolves. This will create a simple syrup. Take it out from heat and let it cool.

2. Once the simple syrup has cooled, add one cup of freshly squeezed lemon juice and the zest of 2 lemons to the syrup. Mix sufficiently.

3. Add a pinch of salt to the lemon mixture and stir until fully incorporated.

4. Pour the lemon mixture into an ice cream maker and churn according to the manufacturer's instructions. This typically takes about 20-25 minutes.

5. During the last few minutes of churning, you can add lemon slices if desired, allowing them to incorporate into the sorbet.

6. Once the sorbet has reached a firm, ice-cream-like consistency, transfer it to an airtight container.

7. Cover the container and freeze the lemon sorbet for at least 3 hours or until it's firm enough to scoop.

8. Before serving, let the sorbet sit at room temperature for a few minutes to soften slightly, making it easier to scoop.

9. Garnish with lemon slices and fresh mint leaves, if desired.

Nutritional Information (per serving, without optional garnishes):

- Carbs: 42 grams

- Fats: 0 grams

- Fiber: 0 grams

- Protein: 0 grams

Poached Pears in Red Wine

Prep Time: 15 minutes
Cook Time: 30 minutes
Number of Servings: 4

Ingredients:

- 4 ripe pears, peeled, halved, and cored
- 1 bottle (750 ml) red wine (such as Merlot or Cabernet Sauvignon)
- 1 cup granulated sugar
- 1 cinnamon stick
- 4 cloves
- 1 strip of orange peel (use a vegetable peeler)
- 1 strip of lemon peel (use a vegetable peeler)
- 1 teaspoon vanilla extract
- Vanilla ice cream or whipped cream for serving (optional)

Instructions:

1. In a large saucepan, add 1 bottle (750 ml) of red wine, one cup of granulated sugar, 1 cinnamon stick, 4 cloves, 1 strip of orange peel, and 1 strip of lemon peel.

2. Heat the mixture over medium heat, stirring until the sugar dissolves and the wine begins to simmer.

3. Once the wine is simmering, add the peeled, halved, and cored pears to the saucepan.

4. Cover the pears with a piece of parchment paper to help keep them submerged in the wine mixture.

5. Allow the pears to simmer in the wine for about 20-30 minutes, or until tender but not mushy. The cooking time may vary depending on the ripeness of the pears.

6. Once the pears are cooked to your liking, use a slotted spoon to carefully take them out from the wine and set them aside.

7. Continue to simmer the red wine mixture until it reduces and thickens into a syrup-like consistency. This should take about 10-15 minutes.

8. Take out the saucepan from heat, discard the cinnamon stick, cloves, and citrus peels, and stir in one teaspoon of vanilla extract.

9. Allow the red wine syrup to cool slightly.

10. Serve each poached pear with a drizzle of the red wine syrup. You can also serve them with vanilla ice cream or whipped cream, if desired.

Nutritional Information (per serving, without optional toppings):

- Carbs: 60 grams

- Fats: 0 grams

- Fiber: 5 grams

- Protein: 1 gram

Almond Flour Brownies

Prep Time: 15 minutes
Cook Time: 25 minutes
Number of Servings: 12

Ingredients:

- 1 1/2 cups almond flour

- 1/2 cup unsweetened cocoa powder

- 1/2 teaspoon baking powder

- 1/4 teaspoon salt

- 1/2 cup unsalted butter, melted

- 1 cup granulated sugar

- 2 large eggs

- 1 teaspoon pure vanilla extract

- 1/2 cup semisweet chocolate chips

Instructions:

1. Turn on your oven and set it to 350°F (175°C) to preheat. Grease an 8x8-inch (20x20 cm) baking pan and line it with parchment paper for easy removal.

2. In a mixing bowl, whisk 1 1/2 cups of almond flour, 1/2 cup of unsweetened cocoa powder, 1/2 teaspoon of baking powder, and 1/4 teaspoon of salt until well combined.

3. In a separate bowl, add 1/2 cup of melted unsalted butter and one cup of granulated sugar. Mix until the sugar is fully incorporated into the melted butter.

4. Add 2 large eggs and one teaspoon of pure vanilla extract to the butter and sugar mixture. Stir until the eggs are well incorporated.

5. Gradually add the dry almond flour and cocoa powder mixture to the wet ingredients. Mix until you have a smooth brownie batter.

6. Fold in 1/2 cup of semisweet chocolate chips into the brownie batter.

7. Pour the brownie batter into the prepared baking pan and spread it out evenly.

8. Bake in the preheated oven for about 25 minutes, or until a toothpick inserted into the center comes out with a few moist crumbs but no wet batter.

9. Take out the brownies from the oven and allow them to cool in the pan for about 10-15 minutes.

10. After cooling in the pan, use the parchment paper to lift the brownies out and transfer them to a wire rack to cool completely.

11. Once cooled, cut the brownies into 12 squares.

Nutritional Information (per brownie):

- Carbs: 22 grams
- Fats: 15 grams
- Fiber: 3 grams
- Protein: 5 grams

Baked Apples with Cinnamon

Prep Time: 15 minutes
Cook Time: 45 minutes
Number of Servings: 4

Ingredients:

- 4 large apples (such as Granny Smith or Honeycrisp)
- 1/4 cup brown sugar
- 1 teaspoon ground cinnamon
- 1/4 cup chopped walnuts or pecans (optional)
- 2 tablespoons unsalted butter, cut into small cubes
- 1/2 cup apple juice or apple cider

Instructions:

1. Turn on your oven and set it to 375°F (190°C) to preheat.
2. Wash and core 4 large apples, leaving the bottoms intact. You can use an apple corer or a paring knife to take out the cores.
3. In a small bowl, add 1/4 cup of brown sugar and one teaspoon of ground cinnamon.
4. If you're using chopped walnuts or pecans, mix them into the brown sugar and cinnamon mixture.
5. Place the cored apples in a baking dish.
6. Stuff each apple cavity with the brown sugar and cinnamon mixture. Be generous with the filling.
7. Top each stuffed apple with two tablespoons of unsalted butter, placing the butter cubes evenly on top of the filling.
8. Pour 1/2 cup of apple juice or apple cider into the bottom of the baking dish. This will help keep the apples moist and create a delicious sauce.
9. Cover the baking dish with aluminum foil and bake in the preheated oven for about 30 minutes.
10. After 30 minutes, take out the foil and continue baking for an extra 15 minutes or until the apples are tender and the tops are slightly caramelized.
11. Carefully take out the baked apples from the oven and let them cool for a few minutes.

12. Serve the baked apples with a drizzle of the caramelized sauce from the baking dish. You can also pair them with a scoop of vanilla ice cream or a dollop of whipped cream if desired.

Nutritional Information (per serving, without optional toppings):

- Carbs: 43 grams

- Fats: 7 grams

- Fiber: 5 grams

- Protein: 1 gram

Banana Ice Cream

Prep Time: 10 minutes
Freeze Time: 2 hours
Number of Servings: 4

Ingredients:

- 4 ripe bananas

- 2 tablespoons honey or maple syrup (optional)

- 1 teaspoon pure vanilla extract (optional)

- Optional toppings: chopped nuts, chocolate chips, or sliced strawberries

Instructions:

1. Peel 4 ripe bananas and slice them into thin rounds.

2. Place the banana slices in a single layer on a parchment paper-lined baking sheet. Ensure not touching each other.

3. If desired, drizzle two tablespoons of honey or maple syrup and one teaspoon of pure vanilla extract over the banana slices. This step is optional but adds sweetness and flavor.

4. Cover the baking sheet with plastic wrap and place it in the freezer. Freeze the banana slices for at least 2 hours or until completely frozen.

5. Once the banana slices are frozen solid, take them out from the freezer.

6. Transfer the frozen banana slices to a food processor or a high-powered blender. If using a blender, you may need to scrape down the sides periodically.

7. Blend the frozen banana slices until they become creamy and smooth. This process may take a few minutes and may require some patience. If the mixture seems too thick, you can add a splash of milk to help it blend.

8. Once the banana mixture has a smooth ice cream-like consistency, it's ready to serve.

9. You can enjoy the banana ice cream as is or add your favorite toppings like chopped nuts, chocolate chips, or sliced strawberries.

10. Serve immediately for a soft-serve texture, or transfer the banana ice cream to an airtight container and freeze for a firmer consistency.

Nutritional Information (per serving, without optional toppings):

- Carbs: 27 grams

- Fats: 0 grams

- Fiber: 3 grams

- Protein: 1 gram

Chia Seed Chocolate Mousse

Prep Time: 10 minutes
Chill Time: 2 hours
Number of Servings: 4

Ingredients:

- 1/2 cup chia seeds

- 2 cups unsweetened almond milk

- 1/4 cup unsweetened cocoa powder

- 1/4 cup honey or maple syrup

- 1 teaspoon pure vanilla extract

- A pinch of salt

- Optional toppings: whipped cream and chocolate shavings

Instructions:

1. In a mixing bowl, add 1/2 cup of chia seeds and two cups of unsweetened almond milk. Stir sufficiently to fully incorporate the chia seeds into the milk.

2. Add 1/4 cup of unsweetened cocoa powder to the chia seed mixture. Mix until the cocoa powder is evenly distributed.

3. Stir in 1/4 cup of honey or maple syrup, one teaspoon of pure vanilla extract, and a pinch of salt. Continue to stir until all the ingredients are well combined.

4. Cover the bowl and refrigerate the chia seed mixture for at least 2 hours, or until it thickens to a pudding-like consistency. You can also leave it in the fridge overnight for a thicker texture.

5. After the mixture has set, give it a good stir to break up any clumps and ensure a smooth consistency.

6. Divide the chia seed chocolate mousse into 4 serving glasses or bowls.

7. If desired, top each serving with a dollop of whipped cream and a sprinkle of chocolate shavings.

8. Serve the chia seed chocolate mousse chilled and enjoy!

Nutritional Information (per serving, without optional toppings):

- Carbs: 20 grams

- Fats: 7 grams

- Fiber: 11 grams

- Protein: 5 grams

Coconut Macaroons

Prep Time: 15 minutes
Cook Time: 20 minutes
Number of Servings: 24

Ingredients:

- 3 cups shredded sweetened coconut

- 3/4 cup granulated sugar

- 1/4 cup all-purpose flour

- 1/4 teaspoon salt

- 4 large egg whites

- 1 teaspoon pure vanilla extract

- Optional: 4 ounces of melted semi-sweet or bittersweet chocolate for dipping (not included in nutritional information)

Instructions:

1. Turn on your oven and set it to 325°F (160°C) to preheat. Line two baking sheets with parchment paper.

2. In a mixing bowl, add three cups of shredded sweetened coconut, 3/4 cup of granulated sugar, 1/4 cup of all-purpose flour, and 1/4 teaspoon of salt. Mix these dry ingredients together.

3. In a separate bowl, beat 4 large egg whites until they reach stiff peaks. This may take a few minutes with an electric mixer.

4. Gently fold the stiff egg whites into the dry ingredient mixture. Be careful not to deflate the egg whites completely; you want to maintain some of the fluffiness.

5. Stir in one teaspoon of pure vanilla extract to the mixture, ensuring it's evenly distributed.

6. Using a spoon or cookie scoop, drop rounded tablespoons of the coconut mixture onto the prepared baking sheets. Space them about 1 inch apart.

7. Bake in the preheated oven for approximately 20 minutes, or until the coconut macaroons turn golden brown around the edges.

8. Take out the macaroons from the oven and let them cool on the baking sheets for a few minutes before transferring them to a wire rack to cool completely.

9. If desired, you can melt 4 ounces of semi-sweet or bittersweet chocolate and dip the bottoms of the cooled macaroons into the chocolate. Place them on parchment paper to let the chocolate set.

10. Allow the chocolate to fully harden before storing the coconut macaroons in an airtight container.

Nutritional Information (per macaroon, without chocolate coating):

- Carbs: 11 grams

- Fats: 4 grams

- Fiber: 1 gram

- Protein: 1 gram

Peach Cobbler
Prep Time: 15 minutes
Cook Time: 45 minutes
Number of Servings: 8

Ingredients:

For the Peach Filling:

- 6 cups sliced fresh or canned peaches (drained)

- 1 cup granulated sugar

- 1/4 cup unsalted butter

- 1 teaspoon pure vanilla extract

- 1/2 teaspoon ground cinnamon

- 1/4 teaspoon salt

For the Cobbler Topping:

- 1 cup all-purpose flour

- 1/2 cup granulated sugar

- 1 1/2 teaspoons baking powder

- 1/2 teaspoon salt

- 1/2 cup milk

- 1/4 cup unsalted butter, melted

Instructions:

1. Turn on your oven and set it to 350°F (175°C) to preheat.

2. In a large saucepan, add 6 cups of sliced peaches, one cup of granulated sugar, 1/4 cup of unsalted butter, one teaspoon of pure

vanilla extract, 1/2 teaspoon of ground cinnamon, and 1/4 teaspoon of salt. Cook over medium heat, stirring occasionally, until the sugar and butter melt and the mixture comes to a simmer. Let it simmer for about 5 minutes, then remove it from the heat.

3. In a separate mixing bowl, prepare the cobbler topping. Add one cup of all-purpose flour, 1/2 cup of granulated sugar, 1 1/2 teaspoons of baking powder, and 1/2 teaspoon of salt.

4. Pour in 1/2 cup of milk and 1/4 cup of melted unsalted butter into the dry ingredients. Stir until just combined; do not overmix.

5. Pour the peach filling into a greased 9x13-inch (23x33 cm) baking dish.

6. Spoon the cobbler topping evenly over the peach filling.

7. Place the baking dish in the preheated oven and bake for approximately 45 minutes, or until the cobbler topping is golden brown and the peach filling is bubbly.

8. Take out the peach cobbler from the oven and let it cool slightly before serving.

9. Serve the warm peach cobbler on its own or with a scoop of vanilla ice cream, if desired.

Nutritional Information (per serving):

- Carbs: 58 grams

- Fats: 14 grams

- Fiber: 3 grams

- Protein: 4 grams

BEVERAGES

Iced Lavender Lemonade Recipe

Prep Time: 10 minutes
Cook Time: 0 minutes
Number of Servings: 4

Ingredients:

- 1/4 cup dried lavender buds
- 1 cup boiling water
- 1/2 cup fresh lemon juice (about 4 lemons)
- 1/2 cup granulated sugar
- 4 cups cold water
- Ice cubes
- Lemon slices and fresh lavender sprigs for garnish (optional)

Instructions:

1. In a heatproof bowl, add the dried lavender buds and one cup of boiling water. Let it steep for about 5 minutes to make lavender tea. Strain the tea to take out the lavender buds and let it cool to room temperature.

2. In a separate bowl, mix the fresh lemon juice and granulated sugar until the sugar is completely dissolved, creating a lemon syrup.

3. In a large pitcher, add the lavender tea, lemon syrup, and 4 cups of cold water. Stir sufficiently to ensure everything is thoroughly mixed.

4. Fill serving glasses with ice cubes.

5. Pour the lavender lemonade over the ice cubes, filling each glass about two-thirds full.

6. Garnish with lemon slices and fresh lavender sprigs if desired.

7. Serve the iced lavender lemonade immediately and enjoy!

Nutritional Information (per serving):

- Carbs: 25g

- Fats: 0g

- Fiber: 0g

- Protein: 0g

Minty Cucumber Water Recipe

Prep Time: 10 minutes
Cook Time: 0 minutes
Number of Servings: 4

Ingredients:

- 1 large cucumber, thinly sliced

- 1/4 cup fresh mint leaves

- 1 lemon, thinly sliced

- 4 cups cold water

- Ice cubes

Instructions:

1. In a large pitcher, add the thinly sliced cucumber, fresh mint leaves, and lemon slices.

2. Gently muddle the ingredients in the pitcher using a muddler or the back of a spoon. This will release the flavors from the cucumber, mint, and lemon.

3. Add 4 cups of cold water to the pitcher and stir sufficiently.

4. Fill serving glasses with ice cubes.

5. Pour the minty cucumber water over the ice cubes, filling each glass.

6. Optionally, garnish with additional mint leaves or cucumber slices for a fresh touch.

7. Serve the minty cucumber water immediately and enjoy!

Nutritional Information (per serving):

- Carbs: 4g

- Fats: 0g

- Fiber: 1g
- Protein: 0g

Hibiscus Tea with Stevia Recipe

Prep Time: 5 minutes
Cook Time: 10 minutes
Number of Servings: 4

Ingredients:

- 4 cups water
- 1/2 cup dried hibiscus petals
- 1/4 cup stevia leaves or 8-10 stevia packets (adjust to taste)
- Ice cubes (optional)
- Lemon or lime slices for garnish (optional)

Instructions:

1. In a medium saucepan, bring 4 cups of water to a boil.
2. Once the water is boiling, add the dried hibiscus petals to the saucepan.
3. Reduce the heat to low and let the hibiscus petals simmer for 10 minutes. This will create a strong hibiscus tea.
4. After simmering, take out the saucepan from heat and let it cool for a few minutes.
5. While the tea is still warm, add the stevia leaves or stevia packets to the saucepan. Stir to dissolve the stevia. Adjust the amount of stevia to your desired level of sweetness.
6. Allow the hibiscus tea to cool to room temperature.
7. Strain the tea to take out the hibiscus petals and any remaining stevia leaves.
8. If desired, add ice cubes to serving glasses.
9. Pour the hibiscus tea over the ice cubes.
10. Optionally, garnish with lemon or lime slices for added flavor and presentation.

11. Serve the hibiscus tea with stevia immediately, or refrigerate for a refreshing cold drink.

Nutritional Information (per serving):

- Carbs: 2g

- Fats: 0g

- Fiber: 0g

- Protein: 0g

Golden Milk Latte Recipe

Prep Time: 5 minutes
Cook Time: 10 minutes
Number of Servings: 2

Ingredients:

- 2 cups unsweetened almond milk

- 1 teaspoon ground turmeric

- 1/2 teaspoon ground cinnamon

- 1/4 teaspoon ground ginger

- 1/4 teaspoon ground black pepper

- 1/4 teaspoon ground cardamom

- 1/4 teaspoon ground cloves

- 2 tablespoons honey or maple syrup (adjust to taste)

- 1 teaspoon coconut oil

- 1 teaspoon vanilla extract

Instructions:

1. In a small saucepan, add the unsweetened almond milk, ground turmeric, ground cinnamon, ground ginger, ground black pepper, ground cardamom, and ground cloves.

2. Whisk the mixture to combine the spices evenly with the almond milk.

3. Place the saucepan over medium heat and heat the mixture until it's just about to simmer. Do not let it come to a boil.

4. Reduce the heat to low and let the spiced almond milk simmer gently for about 5-7 minutes, allowing the flavors to meld.

5. Stir in the honey or maple syrup to sweeten the golden milk latte, adjusting the amount to your taste.

6. Add the coconut oil and vanilla extract to the saucepan and stir until the oil is fully incorporated.

7. Take out the saucepan from heat and let it cool slightly.

8. Strain the golden milk latte through a fine-mesh sieve into serving mugs to remove any spice residue.

9. Serve the golden milk latte warm and enjoy the soothing flavors.

Nutritional Information (per serving):

- Carbs: 12g
- Fats: 5g
- Fiber: 1g
- Protein: 1g

Kiwi and Lime Smoothie Recipe

Prep Time: 5 minutes
Cook Time: 0 minutes
Number of Servings: 2

Ingredients:

- 4 ripe kiwis, peeled and sliced
- Juice of 2 limes
- 1 cup plain Greek yogurt
- 1/2 cup almond milk
- 2 tablespoons honey or maple syrup (adjust to taste)
- 1 cup ice cubes

Instructions:

1. Place the peeled and sliced kiwis in a blender.

2. Add the juice of 2 limes to the blender.

3. Spoon in one cup of plain Greek yogurt.

4. Pour in 1/2 cup of almond milk.

5. Add two tablespoons of honey or maple syrup to sweeten the smoothie, adjusting the amount to your taste preference.

6. Drop in one cup of ice cubes to make the smoothie cold and refreshing.

7. Blend all the ingredients together until the mixture is smooth and creamy. If needed, you can add a little more almond milk to achieve your desired consistency.

8. Once blended, taste the smoothie and adjust the sweetness or tartness by adding more honey, lime juice, or kiwi if necessary.

9. Pour the kiwi and lime smoothie into glasses.

10. Serve the smoothie immediately and enjoy this tangy and refreshing treat!

Nutritional Information (per serving):

*   Carbs: 34g

*   Fats: 2g

*   Fiber: 4g

*   Protein: 7g

Ginger Turmeric Infused Water Recipe

Prep Time: 5 minutes
Cook Time: 0 minutes
Number of Servings: 4

Ingredients:

*   4 cups water

*   1-inch piece of fresh ginger, thinly sliced

*   1-inch piece of fresh turmeric, thinly sliced

- 1 lemon, thinly sliced

- Honey or maple syrup (optional, to taste)

Instructions:

1. In a large pitcher, add 4 cups of water.

2. Add the thinly sliced fresh ginger to the water.

3. Add the thinly sliced fresh turmeric to the pitcher.

4. Include the thinly sliced lemon rounds in the pitcher as well.

5. If desired, you can add honey or maple syrup to sweeten the infused water. Start with 1-2 tablespoons and adjust to your taste preference. Note that this step is optional, and you can leave the water unsweetened if you prefer.

6. Stir the ingredients gently to distribute the flavors.

7. Allow the ginger turmeric infused water to sit for at least 30 minutes at room temperature to let the flavors infuse.

8. After infusing, you can serve the water immediately or refrigerate it to enjoy it cold.

9. Pour the infused water into glasses or use a pitcher with a strainer to prevent ginger, turmeric, and lemon slices from being poured into the glasses.

10. Serve the ginger turmeric infused water and stay refreshed!

Nutritional Information (per serving):

- Carbs: 2g

- Fats: 0g

- Fiber: 0g

- Protein: 0g

Raspberry Almond Milkshake Recipe
Prep Time: 5 minutes
Cook Time: 0 minutes
Number of Servings: 2

Ingredients:

- 2 cups frozen raspberries
- 2 cups almond milk
- 2 tablespoons almond butter
- 2 tablespoons honey or maple syrup (adjust to taste)
- 1 teaspoon vanilla extract
- Ice cubes (optional)

Instructions:

1. In a blender, add two cups of frozen raspberries.
2. Pour in two cups of almond milk.
3. Add two tablespoons of almond butter to the blender.
4. Sweeten the milkshake with two tablespoons of honey or maple syrup, adjusting the amount to your preferred level of sweetness.
5. Include one teaspoon of vanilla extract for added flavor.
6. If you want a thicker consistency or a colder shake, you can add a handful of ice cubes to the blender.
7. Blend all the ingredients until the mixture is smooth and creamy. If it's too thick, you can add more almond milk to reach your desired consistency.
8. Taste the milkshake and adjust the sweetness if necessary by adding more honey or maple syrup.
9. Once blended to your satisfaction, pour the raspberry almond milkshake into glasses.
10. Serve the milkshake immediately for a refreshing and delicious treat!

Nutritional Information (per serving):

- Carbs: 30g
- Fats: 13g
- Fiber: 10g
- Protein: 4g

Blueberry Basil Lemonade Recipe

Prep Time: 15 minutes
Cook Time: 0 minutes
Number of Servings: 4

Ingredients:

- 1 cup fresh blueberries
- 1/4 cup fresh basil leaves
- 1 cup freshly squeezed lemon juice (about 6-8 lemons)
- 1/2 cup granulated sugar
- 4 cups cold water
- Ice cubes
- Lemon slices and fresh basil sprigs for garnish (optional)

Instructions:

1. In a blender, add one cup of fresh blueberries.
2. Add 1/4 cup of fresh basil leaves to the blender.
3. Blend the blueberries and basil until you have a smooth puree.
4. Strain the blueberry-basil puree through a fine-mesh sieve into a large pitcher to remove any solids. You should have about 1/2 cup of the puree.
5. In the same pitcher, add one cup of freshly squeezed lemon juice.
6. Stir in 1/2 cup of granulated sugar to sweeten the lemonade.
7. Add 4 cups of cold water to the pitcher and mix sufficiently to combine all the ingredients.
8. Fill serving glasses with ice cubes.
9. Pour the blueberry basil lemonade over the ice cubes, filling each glass.
10. Optionally, garnish with lemon slices and fresh basil sprigs for a lovely presentation.
11. Serve the blueberry basil lemonade immediately and enjoy!

Nutritional Information (per serving):

- Carbs: 32g

- Fats: 0g

- Fiber: 1g

- Protein: 0g

Peach and Coconut Water Smoothie Recipe

Prep Time: 5 minutes
Cook Time: 0 minutes
Number of Servings: 2

Ingredients:

- 2 ripe peaches, pitted and sliced

- 1 cup coconut water

- 1/2 cup Greek yogurt

- 2 tablespoons honey or maple syrup (adjust to taste)

- 1/2 teaspoon vanilla extract

- Ice cubes (optional)

Instructions:

1. In a blender, place the sliced and pitted ripe peaches.

2. Pour in one cup of coconut water.

3. Add 1/2 cup of Greek yogurt to the blender.

4. Sweeten the smoothie with two tablespoons of honey or maple syrup, adjusting the amount to your desired level of sweetness.

5. Include 1/2 teaspoon of vanilla extract for added flavor.

6. If you prefer a colder or thicker smoothie, you can add a handful of ice cubes to the blender.

7. Blend all the ingredients until the mixture is smooth and creamy. If the smoothie is too thick, you can add more coconut water to reach your desired consistency.

8. Taste the smoothie and adjust the sweetness if necessary by adding more honey or maple syrup.

9. Once blended to your liking, pour the peach and coconut water smoothie into glasses.

10. Serve the smoothie immediately for a refreshing and tropical treat!

Nutritional Information (per serving):

- Carbs: 27g

- Fats: 1g

- Fiber: 2g

- Protein: 5g

Matcha Green Tea Latte Recipe
Prep Time: 5 minutes
Cook Time: 5 minutes
Number of Servings: 2

Ingredients:

- 2 teaspoons matcha green tea powder

- 2 cups milk (dairy or plant-based)

- 2 tablespoons honey or maple syrup (adjust to taste)

- 1/2 teaspoon vanilla extract

- Hot water (for frothing)

Instructions:

1. In a small bowl, add two teaspoons of matcha green tea powder.

2. Heat two cups of milk in a saucepan over medium heat until it's hot but not boiling. Be sure to whisk it occasionally to prevent scalding.

3. While the milk is heating, add two tablespoons of honey or maple syrup to the matcha powder. You can adjust the sweetness to your preference.

4. Pour in 1/2 teaspoon of vanilla extract into the matcha mixture.

5. Add a small amount of hot water (about two tablespoons) to the matcha mixture. Use a bamboo whisk or a small whisk to mix the ingredients into a smooth paste.

6. Once the milk is hot, remove it from the heat.

7. Use a milk frother or a whisk to froth the milk until it's nice and foamy.

8. Divide the matcha paste evenly between two serving mugs.

9. Pour the frothed hot milk over the matcha paste in the mugs. Stir sufficiently to combine the matcha with the milk.

10. Serve the matcha green tea latte hot and enjoy!

Nutritional Information (per serving):

- Carbs: 21g

- Fats: 4g

- Fiber: 1g

- Protein: 6g

Ginger Mint Tea Recipe

Prep Time: 5 minutes
Cook Time: 10 minutes
Number of Servings: 2

Ingredients:

- 2 cups water

- 1-inch piece of fresh ginger, sliced

- 1/4 cup fresh mint leaves

- 2 tablespoons honey or maple syrup (adjust to taste)

- Lemon slices (optional, for garnish)

Instructions:

1. In a small saucepan, bring two cups of water to a boil.

2. While the water is heating, slice a 1-inch piece of fresh ginger.

3. Once the water is boiling, add the sliced ginger to the saucepan.

4. Reduce the heat to low and let the ginger simmer in the water for about 10 minutes. This will infuse the water with the ginger's flavor.

KATHLEEN H. JENSEN

5. After simmering, take out the saucepan from heat.

6. Add 1/4 cup of fresh mint leaves to the saucepan.

7. Cover the saucepan and let the mint steep in the ginger-infused water for 5 minutes.

8. Strain the ginger mint tea to take out the ginger slices and mint leaves. This will leave you with a clear tea.

9. Sweeten the tea with two tablespoons of honey or maple syrup, adjusting the amount to your desired level of sweetness.

10. If desired, garnish with lemon slices for extra flavor.

11. Serve the ginger mint tea hot and savor the soothing blend of flavors.

Nutritional Information (per serving):

- Carbs: 17g

- Fats: 0g

- Fiber: 0g

- Protein: 0g

Cucumber Lemonade Recipe

Prep Time: 10 minutes
Cook Time: 0 minutes
Number of Servings: 4

Ingredients:

- 2 cucumbers, peeled and sliced

- 1 cup fresh lemon juice (about 8 lemons)

- 1/2 cup granulated sugar

- 4 cups cold water

- Ice cubes

- Lemon slices and cucumber slices for garnish (optional)

Instructions:

1. Begin by peeling and slicing 2 cucumbers.

2. In a blender, place the peeled and sliced cucumbers.

3. Squeeze one cup of fresh lemon juice from approximately 8 lemons.

4. Add 1/2 cup of granulated sugar to the blender to sweeten the lemonade.

5. Pour in 4 cups of cold water.

6. Blend the mixture until it's smooth and all the ingredients are well combined.

7. Taste the cucumber lemonade and adjust the sweetness or tartness by adding more sugar or lemon juice if needed.

8. Fill serving glasses with ice cubes.

9. Pour the cucumber lemonade over the ice cubes, filling each glass.

10. Optionally, garnish with lemon slices and cucumber slices for a fresh presentation.

11. Serve the cucumber lemonade immediately and enjoy its cool and refreshing flavor!

Nutritional Information (per serving):

- Carbs: 30g

- Fats: 0g

- Fiber: 1g

- Protein: 1g

Almond Milk Hot Chocolate Recipe

Prep Time: 5 minutes
Cook Time: 10 minutes
Number of Servings: 2

Ingredients:

- 2 cups unsweetened almond milk

- 1/4 cup unsweetened cocoa powder

- 2 tablespoons honey or maple syrup (adjust to taste)

- 1/4 teaspoon vanilla extract

- Pinch of salt

- Vegan whipped cream or regular whipped cream (optional, for topping)

Instructions:

1. In a small saucepan, add two cups of unsweetened almond milk.

2. Whisk in 1/4 cup of unsweetened cocoa powder to the almond milk.

3. Heat the mixture over medium heat, stirring constantly until it's hot but not boiling.

4. Once the mixture is hot, add two tablespoons of honey or maple syrup to sweeten the hot chocolate, adjusting the amount to your preferred level of sweetness.

5. Stir in 1/4 teaspoon of vanilla extract for added flavor.

6. Add a pinch of salt to enhance the chocolate flavor. Stir sufficiently to combine.

7. Continue to heat the hot chocolate for about 2-3 more minutes, ensuring it's well mixed and heated through.

8. Once heated, take out the saucepan from the heat.

9. Pour the almond milk hot chocolate into serving mugs.

10. If desired, top with vegan whipped cream or regular whipped cream for an extra indulgent touch.

11. Serve the almond milk hot chocolate immediately and savor the warm and comforting flavors!

Nutritional Information (per serving):

- Carbs: 19g

- Fats: 6g

- Fiber: 5g

- Protein: 3g

Blueberry Lavender Infused Water Recipe

Prep Time: 5 minutes
Cook Time: 0 minutes
Number of Servings: 4

Ingredients:

- 1 cup fresh blueberries
- 2 tablespoons dried lavender buds
- 4 cups water
- Ice cubes (optional)
- Lemon slices and fresh lavender sprigs for garnish (optional)

Instructions:

1. Begin by rinsing one cup of fresh blueberries under cold running water.
2. In a pitcher, place the rinsed blueberries.
3. Add two tablespoons of dried lavender buds to the pitcher with the blueberries.
4. Pour in 4 cups of water over the blueberries and lavender.
5. If you prefer a colder infused water, you can add ice cubes to the pitcher.
6. Gently stir the ingredients to combine them, releasing the flavors of the blueberries and lavender.
7. Allow the infused water to sit for at least 30 minutes at room temperature to let the flavors meld.
8. Optionally, garnish the individual glasses with lemon slices and fresh lavender sprigs for added flavor and presentation.
9. Serve the blueberry lavender infused water and enjoy its delightful taste and aroma!

Nutritional Information (per serving):

- Carbs: 8g
- Fats: 0g

- Fiber: 2g

- Protein: 0g

Iced Chamomile Tea Recipe

Prep Time: 5 minutes
Cook Time: 0 minutes
Number of Servings: 4

Ingredients:

- 4 chamomile tea bags

- 4 cups boiling water

- 2 tablespoons honey or maple syrup (adjust to taste)

- 1 lemon, thinly sliced

- Ice cubes

- Fresh mint leaves for garnish (optional)

Instructions:

1. Start by boiling 4 cups of water in a kettle or saucepan.

2. In a heatproof pitcher or container, place 4 chamomile tea bags.

3. Pour the freshly boiled water over the chamomile tea bags.

4. Allow the tea bags to steep in the hot water for about 5 minutes or until you reach your desired strength of chamomile flavor.

5. After steeping, take out the tea bags from the hot water and discard them.

6. Sweeten the chamomile tea with two tablespoons of honey or maple syrup, adjusting the amount to your taste preference.

7. Thinly slice 1 lemon and add the lemon slices to the chamomile tea. This will infuse a gentle citrus flavor.

8. Let the tea cool to room temperature, then refrigerate it until chilled.

9. Fill serving glasses with ice cubes.

10. Pour the chilled chamomile tea over the ice cubes, filling each glass.

11. Optionally, garnish with fresh mint leaves for added aroma and presentation.

12. Serve the iced chamomile tea and enjoy its soothing and refreshing qualities!

Nutritional Information (per serving):

- Carbs: 11g

- Fats: 0g

- Fiber: 0g

- Protein: 0g

Strawberry Banana Smoothie Recipe

Prep Time: 5 minutes
Cook Time: 0 minutes
Number of Servings: 2

Ingredients:

- 1 cup fresh or frozen strawberries

- 2 ripe bananas, peeled and sliced

- 1 cup plain Greek yogurt

- 1/2 cup almond milk

- 2 tablespoons honey or maple syrup (adjust to taste)

- Ice cubes (optional)

Instructions:

1. Begin by preparing the fruit. If you are using fresh strawberries, wash and hull them. If you are using frozen strawberries, there is no need to wash them.

2. In a blender, place one cup of fresh or frozen strawberries.

3. Add 2 ripe bananas to the blender. Ensure peeled and sliced for easier blending.

4. Spoon in one cup of plain Greek yogurt.

5. Pour in 1/2 cup of almond milk.

6. Sweeten the smoothie with two tablespoons of honey or maple syrup, adjusting the amount to your preferred level of sweetness.

7. If you prefer a colder and thicker smoothie, you can add a handful of ice cubes to the blender.

8. Blend all the ingredients until the mixture is smooth and creamy. If it's too thick, you can add more almond milk to achieve your desired consistency.

9. Taste the smoothie and adjust the sweetness if necessary by adding more honey or maple syrup.

10. Once blended to your satisfaction, pour the strawberry banana smoothie into glasses.

11. Serve the smoothie immediately for a refreshing and fruity treat!

Nutritional Information (per serving):

- Carbs: 38g

- Fats: 2g

- Fiber: 4g

- Protein: 9g

Turmeric Latte Recipe

Prep Time: 5 minutes
Cook Time: 10 minutes
Number of Servings: 2

Ingredients:

- 2 cups milk (dairy or plant-based)

- 1 teaspoon ground turmeric

- 1/2 teaspoon ground cinnamon

- 1/4 teaspoon ground ginger

- 1/4 teaspoon ground cardamom

- 2 tablespoons honey or maple syrup (adjust to taste)

- 1/2 teaspoon vanilla extract

- A pinch of black pepper (optional)
- Ground cinnamon or turmeric for garnish (optional)

Instructions:

1. In a small saucepan, add two cups of milk (dairy or plant-based). Heat it over medium-low heat, stirring occasionally, until it's hot but not boiling.

2. While the milk is heating, gather your spices. You'll need one teaspoon of ground turmeric, 1/2 teaspoon of ground cinnamon, 1/4 teaspoon of ground ginger, and 1/4 teaspoon of ground cardamom.

3. Once the milk is hot, whisk in the ground turmeric, ground cinnamon, ground ginger, and ground cardamom. Continue to heat the milk while stirring for about 2-3 more minutes to infuse the flavors.

4. Add two tablespoons of honey or maple syrup to sweeten the turmeric latte, adjusting the amount to your desired level of sweetness.

5. Stir in 1/2 teaspoon of vanilla extract for added flavor.

6. If you like, add a pinch of black pepper to enhance the absorption of curcumin (the active compound in turmeric). This step is optional but recommended.

7. Continue to heat the turmeric latte for another 2-3 minutes, ensuring all the ingredients are well combined.

8. Take out the saucepan from heat.

9. Pour the turmeric latte into serving mugs.

10. Optionally, garnish with a sprinkle of ground cinnamon or turmeric for extra flavor and a lovely presentation.

11. Serve the turmeric latte hot and savor its soothing and aromatic qualities!

Nutritional Information (per serving):

- Carbs: 27g
- Fats: 4g

- Fiber: 1g

- Protein: 5g

Carrot and Orange Juice Recipe

Prep Time: 10 minutes
Cook Time: 0 minutes
Number of Servings: 2

Ingredients:

- 4 large carrots, peeled and sliced

- 4 large oranges, peeled and segmented

- 1/2 cup water

- 2 tablespoons honey or maple syrup (adjust to taste)

- Ice cubes (optional)

- Orange slices and carrot sticks for garnish (optional)

Instructions:

1. Begin by preparing the carrots. Peel and slice 4 large carrots.

2. Peel and segment 4 large oranges, removing any seeds if present.

3. In a blender, place the sliced carrots.

4. Add the segmented oranges to the blender.

5. Pour in 1/2 cup of water to help with blending.

6. Sweeten the juice with two tablespoons of honey or maple syrup, adjusting the amount to your desired level of sweetness.

7. If you prefer a colder juice, you can add ice cubes to the blender.

8. Blend all the ingredients until you have a smooth and well-mixed juice. If necessary, you can add more water to achieve your desired consistency.

9. Taste the carrot and orange juice and adjust the sweetness if needed by adding more honey or maple syrup.

10. Once blended to your satisfaction, pour the juice into glasses.

11. Optionally, garnish with orange slices and carrot sticks for a fresh and colorful presentation.

12. Serve the carrot and orange juice immediately for a nutritious and refreshing beverage!

Nutritional Information (per serving):

- Carbs: 45g

- Fats: 0g

- Fiber: 7g

- Protein: 3g

Pineapple Coconut Water Recipe
Prep Time: 10 minutes
Cook Time: 0 minutes
Number of Servings: 4

Ingredients:

- 2 cups fresh pineapple chunks

- 4 cups coconut water

- 2 tablespoons honey or maple syrup (adjust to taste)

- Ice cubes

- Fresh pineapple slices for garnish (optional)

- Fresh mint leaves for garnish (optional)

Instructions:

1. Start by preparing two cups of fresh pineapple chunks. You can use a ripe pineapple and cut it into bite-sized pieces.

2. In a pitcher, place the fresh pineapple chunks.

3. Pour in 4 cups of coconut water over the pineapple. You can use coconut water from a carton or freshly extracted coconut water.

4. Sweeten the pineapple coconut water with two tablespoons of honey or maple syrup, adjusting the amount to your preferred level of sweetness.

5. If you prefer a colder drink, you can add ice cubes to the pitcher.

6. Stir the ingredients well to combine and let the flavors meld for a few minutes.

7. Optionally, garnish individual glasses with fresh pineapple slices and a few fresh mint leaves for added flavor and presentation.

8. Serve the pineapple coconut water immediately for a tropical and hydrating refreshment!

Nutritional Information (per serving):

- Carbs: 24g

- Fats: 0g

- Fiber: 2g

- Protein: 1g

Chapter 10

30-Day Meal Plan

Week 1

Day 1

- **Breakfast:** Quinoa Breakfast Bowl with Berries
- **Lunch:** Lemon Dill Potato Soup
- **Dinner:** Lemon Herb Baked Tilapia

Day 2

- **Breakfast:** Sweet Potato and Spinach Breakfast Skillet
- **Lunch:** Creamy Parsnip and Apple Soup
- **Dinner:** Balsamic Glazed Chicken Thighs

Day 3

- **Breakfast:** Green Smoothie Bowl with Almond Butter
- **Lunch:** Thai Coconut Shrimp Soup
- **Dinner:** Stuffed Portobello Mushrooms with Quinoa

Day 4

- **Breakfast:** Cinnamon Oatmeal with Walnuts
- **Lunch:** White Bean and Kale Soup
- **Dinner:** Turkey and Zucchini Meatballs

Day 5

- **Breakfast:** Chia Seed Pudding with Mango
- **Lunch:** Creamy Spinach and Artichoke Soup
- **Dinner:** Baked Cod with Lemon Dill Sauce

Day 6

- **Breakfast:** Veggie Breakfast Tacos with Avocado

- **Lunch:** Cucumber Gazpacho
- **Dinner:** Tofu and Vegetable Stir-Fry with Teriyaki Sauce

Day 7

- **Breakfast:** Pumpkin Spice Overnight Oats
- **Lunch:** Roasted Garlic and Potato Soup
- **Dinner:** Roasted Duck Breast with Orange Glaze

Week 2

Day 8

- **Breakfast:** Broccoli and Feta Breakfast Muffins
- **Lunch:** Moroccan Lentil Soup
- **Dinner:** Beef and Broccoli Stir-Fry

Day 9

- **Breakfast:** Pumpkin Spice Chia Pudding
- **Lunch:** Creamy Tomato and Red Pepper Soup
- **Dinner:** Chicken Piccata with Capers

Day 10

- **Breakfast:** Spinach and Mushroom Breakfast Casserole
- **Lunch:** Chicken and Rice Congee
- **Dinner:** Lemon Herb Grilled Chicken

Day 11

- **Breakfast:** Coconut Flour Waffles with Mixed Berry Compote
- **Lunch:** Creamy Carrot Soup
- **Dinner:** Beef Stroganoff

Day 12

- **Breakfast:** Turmeric and Ginger Oatmeal
- **Lunch:** Potato Leek Soup

- **Dinner:** Stuffed Bell Peppers with Ground Turkey

Day 13

- **Breakfast:** Broccoli and Smoked Salmon Egg Muffins
- **Lunch:** Butternut Squash Bisque
- **Dinner:** Grilled Shrimp with Garlic Butter

Day 14

- **Breakfast:** Turmeric and Ginger Breakfast Quinoa Bowl
- **Lunch:** Tomato Basil Soup
- **Dinner:** Eggplant Parmesan

Week 3

Day 15

- **Breakfast:** Spinach and Feta Egg White Omelette
- **Lunch:** Creamy Mushroom Soup
- **Dinner:** Tofu Stir-Fry with Ginger Sauce

Day 16

- **Breakfast:** Lemon Dill Potato Soup
- **Lunch:** Creamed Cauliflower Recipe
- **Dinner:** Pork Tenderloin with Apples

Day 17

- **Breakfast:** Radicchio and Orange Salad
- **Lunch:** Lemon Garlic Roasted Broccolini Recipe
- **Dinner:** Baked Cod with Herbs

Day 18

- **Breakfast:** Roasted Eggplant and Tomato Salad
- **Lunch:** Miso Glazed Eggplant Recipe
- **Dinner:** Zucchini Noodles with Pesto

Day 19

- **Breakfast:** Tuna and Avocado Salad
- **Lunch:** Ginger Soy Glazed Carrots Recipe
- **Dinner:** Lemon Herb Baked Tilapia

Day 20

- **Breakfast:** Jicama and Mango Salad
- **Lunch:** Creamy Polenta Cakes Recipe
- **Dinner:** Balsamic Glazed Chicken Thighs

Day 21

- **Breakfast:** Red Cabbage Slaw with Lemon Dressing
- **Lunch:** Roasted Buttery Turnips Recipe
- **Dinner:** Stuffed Portobello Mushrooms with Quinoa

Week 4

Day 22

- **Breakfast:** Spinach and Strawberry Salad
- **Lunch:** Parmesan Zucchini Rounds Recipe
- **Dinner:** Tofu and Vegetable Stir-Fry with Teriyaki Sauce

Day 23

- **Breakfast:** Roasted Butternut Squash Salad
- **Lunch:** Cabbage and Bacon Saute Recipe
- **Dinner:** Roasted Duck Breast with Orange Glaze

Day 24

- **Breakfast:** Broccoli and Apple Salad
- **Lunch:** Sautéed Swiss Chard with Lemon Recipe
- **Dinner:** Beef and Broccoli Stir-Fry

Day 25

- **Breakfast:** Beet and Goat Cheese Carpaccio
- **Lunch:** Celeriac and Potato Mash Recipe
- **Dinner:** Chicken Piccata with Capers

Day 26

- **Breakfast:** Cucumber and Red Onion Salad with Yogurt Dressing
- **Lunch:** Mashed Potatoes Recipe
- **Dinner:** Lemon Herb Grilled Chicken

Day 27

- **Breakfast:** Caprese Salad with Balsamic Reduction
- **Lunch:** Garlic Roasted Asparagus Recipe
- **Dinner:** Beef Stroganoff

Day 28

- **Breakfast:** Greek Salad with Feta and Olives
- **Lunch:** Buttery Corn on the Cob Recipe
- **Dinner:** Grilled Shrimp with Garlic Butter

Week 5:

Day 29

- **Breakfast:** Mandarin Orange Spinach Salad
- **Lunch:** Roasted Brussels Sprouts Recipe
- **Dinner:** Eggplant Parmesan

Day 30

- **Breakfast:** Quinoa and Chickpea Salad
- **Lunch:** Glazed Carrots Recipe
- **Dinner:** Zucchini Noodles with Pesto

Chapter 11

Tips for Managing a Low-Fiber Diet Long-term

Although the low-fiber diet is typically recommended as a temporary solution for addressing certain health concerns, some individuals may need to follow this diet longer. Maintaining a low-fiber diet for an extended period requires careful and sustainable planning, whether it's due to a chronic condition or ongoing management of digestive health.

This chapter will discuss the different aspects of managing a low fiber diet in the long term. We'll discuss tips for maintaining nutritional balance, strategies for dining out while adhering to dietary restrictions, and how to prioritize both physical and emotional well-being in the context of your specific nutritional needs. Adopting a long-term low fiber diet doesn't require sacrificing flavor or quality of life. Instead, it involves developing a sustainable and enjoyable eating plan that promotes your overall health.

Tips for dining out

1. Check the restaurant's menu and reviews beforehand to ensure it meets your preferences and expectations.
2. Make a reservation if possible, especially during peak hours, to avoid waiting.

Dining out with friends and family is a joyful experience, and being on a low-fiber diet doesn't have to prevent you from enjoying it.

Here are some strategies to help you maintain your dietary needs while enjoying meals at restaurants:

Research Ahead: Before choosing a restaurant, review their menu online to identify low-fiber options. Numerous establishments provide a diverse range of dishes that can be customized to meet your specific dietary needs.

Communicate Your Needs: Feel free to inform your server about any dietary restrictions you may have. Many restaurants are willing to accommodate special requests, such as preparing dishes without high-fiber ingredients.

Request for Substitutions: Are there any modifications available for dishes to accommodate a low-fiber diet? Request substitutions, such as mashed potatoes as an alternative to a baked potato, or steamed vegetables instead of a salad.

Avoid High-Fiber Foods: Be aware of common high-fiber foods, such as whole grains, beans, and certain vegetables, that may act as triggers for some individuals. Choose dishes that do not contain these ingredients.

Portion Control: Restaurant portions may exceed the recommended size for a low-fiber diet. Consider sharing a dish or requesting a takeout container to enjoy the meal over multiple meals.

Managing Dietary Restrictions

Long-term dietary restrictions can present challenges, both physically and emotionally. Here are some strategies for coping effectively:

Support System: Engage with a support network, such as family, friends, or online communities, that consists of individuals with similar dietary needs. Sharing experiences and tips can provide valuable insights and advice.

Stay Informed: Continuously educate yourself about your medical condition and dietary needs. Having more knowledge about nutrition can help you effectively manage your diet and make well-informed choices.

Regular Check-Ups: It is essential to schedule regular check-ups with your healthcare provider or dietitian. Health professionals can monitor your health and adjust your diet or treatment plan as needed.

Practice mindful eating: To fully enjoy your meals and avoid overeating, practice mindful eating. Appreciate the flavors and textures of your food, even if your options are restricted.

Plan Ahead: Prepare your meals and snacks ahead of time to prevent unexpected dietary challenges. Having a supply of suitable foods on hand can help alleviate stress.

Conclusion

Maintaining Health and Balance

Maintaining a low fiber diet long-term requires a commitment to overall health and well-being.

Here are some ways to help ensure you maintain balance:

Supplements: Depending on your specific condition and dietary restrictions, you may benefit from dietary supplements to help meet your nutrient requirements. Please consult your healthcare provider for further discussion.

Exercise: Regular physical activity can support digestion and contribute to overall health. Consult your healthcare provider for exercise recommendations that align with your specific dietary needs.

Mental Health: Recognize the significant impact of dietary restrictions on your mental health. If you're experiencing emotional difficulties, seeking assistance from a mental health professional is advisable.

Explore and Experiment: Embrace the culinary adventure of a low fiber diet and enjoy the journey. Discovering new recipes, experimenting with different cooking techniques, and incorporating new ingredients can help to make your meals more exciting and pleasurable.

Maintaining a low fiber diet long-term can be a challenging but manageable journey. By implementing effective strategies, having a supportive network, and prioritizing your health and well-being, you can successfully navigate this journey and still find happiness in life, despite any dietary restrictions you may have. This chapter provides guidance on how to make your long-term low fiber diet a sustainable and fulfilling part of your lifestyle.

Recipe Index

Printed in Great Britain
by Amazon